HEAL
YOUR
GUT, SAVE
YOUR
BRAIN

ALSO BY PARTHA NANDI

Ask Dr. Nandi: 5 Steps to Becoming Your Own #HealthHero for Longevity, Well-Being, and a Joyful Life

HEAL YOUR GUT, SAVE YOUR BRAIN

The Five Pillars of Enhancing Your Gut and Optimizing Your Cognitive Health

PARTHA NANDI, M.D.

MAYO CLINIC PRESS

MAYO CLINIC PRESS
200 First St. SW
Rochester, MN 55905
mcpress.mayoclinic.org

The medical information in this book is true and complete to the best of our knowledge. This book is intended only as an informative guide for those wishing to learn more about health issues. It is not intended to replace, countermand or conflict with advice given to you by your own physician. The ultimate decision concerning your care should be made between you and your doctor. Information in this book is offered with no guarantees. The author and publisher disclaim all liability in connection with the use of this book. The views expressed are the author's personal views, and do not necessarily reflect the policy or position of Mayo Clinic.

To stay informed about Mayo Clinic Press, please subscribe to our free e-newsletter at mcpress.mayoclinic.org or follow us on social media.

For bulk sales to employers, member groups and health-related companies, contact Mayo Clinic at SpecialSalesMayoBooks@mayo.edu.

Proceeds from the sale of every book benefit important medical research and education at Mayo Clinic.

The publisher gratefully acknowledges the medical expertise provided by Denise M. Millstine, M.D., and Meredith R. Wicklund, M.D.

Cover design: Nikolaas Eickelbeck
Cover images: dinosoftlabs/iStock/Getty Images Plus via Getty Images | Coquet Adrien/iStock/ Getty Images Plus via Getty Images | verodika/iStock/Getty Images Plus via Getty Images

Library of Congress Cataloging-in-Publication Data
Names: Nandi, Partha, author.
Title: Heal your gut, save your brain : the five pillars of enhancing your gut and optimizing your cognitive health / Partha Nandi.
Description: First edition. | Rochester, MN : Mayo Clinic Press, 2024. | Includes bibliographical references and index. |
Identifiers: LCCN 2024006484 | ISBN 9798887701790 (hardcover) | ISBN 9798887701806 (ebook)
Subjects: LCSH: Brain—Diseases—Nutritional aspects—Popular works. | Brain—Diseases— Prevention—Popular works. | Gastrointestinal system—Microbiology. | Mind and body.
Classification: LCC RC386.2 .N37 2024 | DDC 616.8/04654—dc23/eng/20240509
LC record available at https://lccn.loc.gov/2024006484

ISBN: 979-8-88770-179-0 hardcover
ISBN: 979-8-88770-180-6 ebook

Printed in the U.S.A.

First edition: 2024

CONTENTS

HEAL YOUR GUT, SAVE YOUR BRAIN

INTRODUCTION

One spring evening, my sister and I were having an animated conversation about two political candidates. At one point, our father jumped in and said something matter-of-fact, like, "Listen, they're all the same. It is politics." When he prepared to go to bed, my sister and I returned to our homes. That was the last time we would see Dad as we had always known him.

An hour or so later, my mom called. Dad was slurring his speech, and one side of his mouth was drooping—classic signs of a cerebrovascular accident (CVA, commonly known as a stroke). I rushed back to their house and gave him an aspirin to help thin his blood, and then my sister drove him to the ER, which was only about five minutes away. Although we had managed to get my father to the hospital within thirty minutes of the stroke's onset, the entire left side of his body was paralyzed.

Dad was a brilliant scientist, with a doctorate in polymer chemistry, and a man of many talents. He was an innovative teacher, a mentor to his students, an author, and an inventor. He invented road reflectors, the illuminated stripes we all see at the side of the road that help to keep cars in their lanes even at night. To repair runways during times of war, he developed a substance made of polymers that could be poured into gaping holes, harden in less than thirty minutes, and be stronger than the original surface. He was also an amazing chef, a talented musician, and my first hero.

On the day he had his stroke, Professor Uma Nandi's life changed forever. Our family was shocked, as Dad had looked perfectly well during our visit earlier that evening. Although he had a history of peptic ulcers, he was otherwise healthy, ate a fairly good diet, and took an interest in maintaining his body, mind, and spirit. I could not help but wonder: could we have done anything to prevent this awful event?

SEARCHING FOR ANSWERS

As my family and a team of rehabilitation staff devoted the year after Dad's stroke to nursing him back to health, I could not stop questioning what more he and we could have done to prevent his life-changing and often completely debilitating health crisis. After nearly twenty years as a physician, ten of those spent studying and analyzing the latest research on how gut health affects brain health, I now have the answers I wish I'd had then.

The brain and the gut are neurologically and biochemically connected via millions of nerves and the trillions of microbes that populate the intestines. Known as the gut-brain axis, this communication network between the two systems is vast and complex. Although scientists have known about this axis for some time, the assumption was that the brain controlled how the digestive tract functioned. Only recently has science given the gut its due credit in this relationship. Researchers are learning that the gut microbiome (or microbiota; I will use the terms interchangeably)—the bacteria and other microorganisms (microbes) that naturally live within the intestines and help us digest our food—can influence certain physiological processes in the brain.[1] Our microbiome can have a significant impact on how we think and function—cognition, memory, motor control—for better or worse.

This relationship has come to the forefront of attention as over the past two decades we have seen a rise in stroke (like my dad experienced), Parkinson's disease, and Alzheimer's disease, and a general decline in brain health. In my practice, I regularly see a link between patients' poor gut health and a decline in brain health, and worldwide research supports this link.[2] According to a study done by an international group of neuroscientists, an estimated 25 percent of people who suffer a stroke will develop dementia[3]—a group of symptoms affecting memory, thinking, and social abilities—within one year after their stroke. About 75 percent of people with Parkinson's will develop dementia within ten years from disease onset.[4] And while dementia takes many forms, most people are familiar with Alzheimer's disease, the most common type.

Much of the current research is focused on three leading examples of neurodegeneration (the death of brain cells) that doctors have been struggling to treat effectively: stroke, Alzheimer's, and Parkinson's. Each of these disease states can result in not only neurodegeneration, a progressive loss of brain cells, but also cognitive decline along with a loss of memory and thinking. Furthermore, many recent discoveries highlight the connection between these disorders and well-known risk factors—including genetics, environmental toxins, diabetes, obesity, heart disease, and poor gut health,[5] reinforcing the importance of the connection we are seeing between gut health and brain health.

What gives? What are we doing (or not doing) in our modern lifestyles that is facilitating neurological disorders that lead to cognitive decline? More importantly, what can we do to prevent this decline or at least slow it down? As it turns out, a lot more than you might think. And much of it is as simple as changing basic elements of your lifestyle and the food on your plate.

While this research is becoming more and more accepted in academic circles, it has yet to reach mainstream medicine. Most

HUMAN MICROBIOME PROJECT

From 2007 to 2016, the US National Institutes of Health conducted the Human Microbiome Project, an initiative to characterize gut microbiota and understand their relationship to health and disease.[6] My takeaways (and many other doctors' takeaways) from the project were nothing short of astounding.

- Our microbiome influences our health *as much as or more than* the genes we inherit from our parents.
- Although no two people have identical microbiomes, each of us carries about five hundred different species of microbes in our gut.
- Having a certain combination of microbe species in our microbiome can influence the likelihood of our experiencing a disease such as diabetes.
- Perhaps most importantly, it is likely to change the course of our health by changing our microbiome.

neurologists are not treating neurodegeneration by considering the gut. Although many gastroenterologists find the research interesting, few are applying it in their everyday practices. I am in a minority, and it is my observations, study of the available research, and insights that I share with you here.

BEYOND NUTRITION: THE FIVE PILLARS

Most gut health books offer one solution: nutrition. Some add meditation or exercise to the mix as a way to reduce stress. You are holding the first book on gut health published by a gastroenterologist to offer a holistic solution that combines healing traditions from the East and the West and that often goes well beyond nutrition. This is because every aspect of how we live our lives plays an immense role in how well or poorly our gut functions. The medicines and surgical techniques of Western medicine are critical to adequately addressing gut health, but the science supports the idea that we need to look at additional factors: *movement, purpose, community,* and *spirituality.* While every individual will likely find they need to address one factor more than the others, the research shows that in tandem with nutrition, each of these factors is directly connected to gut health and, therefore, as you'll discover in this work, brain health.[7]

I call these factors the Five Pillars. Let's look at them more closely. Later, we will discuss how each is related to gut and brain health.

Nutrition. We will start with the most straightforward one. When we do not eat healthy and beneficial foods, we do not feel well. Too much of anything—especially sugar, refined flours, and fat—is bound to cause a problem. Of course, as microbiome research and diagnostic tools to detect and measure gut health problems such as irritable bowel syndrome, reflux disease or GERD, lactose intolerance, and digestive disorders in general have advanced, physicians are now better able to pinpoint specific gut issues and prescribe medications along with diet changes and supplements to create balance. While I rely on diagnostic tools as well as medication, I know that if a person is not eating mindfully, with the intention of eating for optimal health, their gut health will be suboptimal.

Movement. This is quite intuitive as well. We have all read the books and articles on the benefits of movement, seen the videos, and experienced the benefits in our lives. The more we exercise, the healthier we are. And it does not have to be a 10K run when a daily twenty-minute walk is often sufficient; it does not have to be powerlifting but can be carrying our groceries from the car instead of having them delivered to our front door. What is especially interesting to me is that our ancestors and even our great-grandparents did not set aside time for fitness; instead, it was incorporated into their daily life. They had fewer conveniences like cars, power tools, and megastores, and so they did things like walk or ride a bike to get where they needed to go, chop wood and sweep the floor, and tend their own garden to grow the foods they ate. That's why I like to think of movement as part of our whole lives, not something separate we do at the gym a few hours a week, focusing on our legs one day and our heart the next.

Purpose. What shapes our lives and provides direction—who we are as human beings, our dreams, our soul's resolve—is our purpose. It is helpful to think about this as part of your legacy. What do you want to leave behind when you are gone? An impressive bank account, or people who remember you for being a wonderful father, compassionate leader, or compelling artist? What your purpose is does not matter as much as the fact that you have one, because not living a purposeful life affects our brains. A recent study at Rush University in Chicago has shown that elderly people with a positive sense of purpose can possibly reduce their cognitive decline by as much as 50 percent.[8] As we will see, such changes affect the gut, and vice versa.

Community. These are your people. Your family, your neighborhood, your circle of friends—those people with whom you celebrate, laugh, cry, and eat lunch. They are the ones you call on for support and the ones who call on *you* for support. Research has shown that the people with the strongest social bonds live the longest.[9] Early and late in life, these tend to be found in wider networks, whereas in the middle of our lives, when we are pulled in more directions—education, career, caring for children and parents—a few deep but meaningful bonds are key. Numerous studies have found a clear connection between social relationships and four markers of health: blood pressure, waist circumference, body mass index, and even gut inflammation.[10] As I will argue in the pages that follow, each relates to our gut and consequently to our brains.

Spirituality. Spirituality is purpose and community turned inward. When we have a spiritual life, we are never alone. Spirituality will look different for each of us, but I see a common denominator: finding our still point in the spinning world, or, to put it in other words, gaining an understanding of our place in the universe. What does that look like for you? It may be a connection with a temple, a mosque, a church, or nature. We often do not think of physical well-being as a direct consequence of our spiritual lives, and so we rarely utter sentences like, "If I take time to meditate, pray, or practice yoga every day, my microbiome will be healthier and that will make my brain healthier." In our culture this is not intuitive, but it can be a powerful insight. We can change a person's diet and see measurable cause and effect, but what science has shown us is that having a spiritual practice diminishes the impact of stressful events in our lives, and when we are less stressed our "fight-or-flight" response is less likely to be triggered—something that is indeed correlated with optimized gut health.[11]

I call the people who frame their lives using the Five Pillars "health heroes." Not only do health heroes take a balanced approach to food and exercise, but they also have a sense of purpose and community, cultivating a meaningful connection to something greater than themselves. Health heroes make body, mind, and spirit their priority, often because an experience with illness has made clear to them the devastation that may befall those who take good health for granted. Health heroes put health first, focusing on prevention and a commitment to the well-being of themselves and others. And, as you will see, a dedication to living as a health hero and strengthening the

ABOUT PROBIOTICS

- Probiotics are the beneficial bacteria that naturally reside in your body, particularly in the gut. These live microorganisms help regulate digestion and intestinal function.
- Each of us has our own, unique microbial environment, kind of like a gut fingerprint, with over a thousand different forms of microorganisms naturally occurring in the body.
- Antibiotics, pregnancy, diet, and other things can mess with your body's natural microbiota, causing a lack of good bacteria.
- When an imbalance in the microbiome occurs, as I've seen in my practice, this can be linked to many other conditions, including arthritis, allergies, and even depression.
- The probiotic bacteria in your system can be restored and sustained by eating fermented foods such as yogurt, kefir, aged cheese, sauerkraut, kimchi, miso, and tempeh, as well as fortified dark chocolate, certain juices, and cereals.
- Probiotics can also be taken as supplements. The two most commonly available strains found in supplements are *Lactobacillus* and *Bifidobacterium*.

Five Pillars can have a direct impact on our well-being when it comes to our gut and brain.

LIVING AS A HEALTH HERO

When one or more of the Five Pillars is forgotten or neglected, our bodies, minds, and lives are out of balance. For years I have been assessing my patients within the framework of the Five Pillars to help them go beyond surviving and progress toward thriving, particularly when it comes to resolving their gut issues.

WHAT DO MEDITATION AND PRAYER HAVE TO DO WITH OUR GUT?

Meditation and prayer have more to do with the gut than you might think. That's because there's a two-way street between mind and gut.

Researchers examining the effects of deep meditation on the gut microbiome structure studied a group of long-term traditional meditators—Tibetan monks. The monks' neighbors, who did not meditate, served as a control group. The researchers found that gut microbiota composition differed between the monks and the control group. Researchers found significantly increased levels of two beneficial types of bacteria (*Megamonas* and *Faecalibacterium*) in the meditators group. Further analysis showed that, in the meditators group, several biochemical pathways—including biosynthesis and metabolism—functioned significantly better. Moreover,

Now that the gut-brain connection is clear to me, I use that framework with the intention of fostering brain health as well. I work with my patients to understand the Five Pillars holistically and determine which of them needs attention.

Take Beverly, for instance. A patient in her fifties, she had recently lost her husband to cancer. Devastated and grieving, she developed severe diarrhea, bloating, cramping, and fatigue. Her symptoms were relentless. I performed diagnostic tests to exclude any serious illnesses and prescribed medicines to help her cope with the symptoms. I also gave her a few simple tips: meditate

plasma levels of substances known to be clinical risk factors for poor gut health, including total cortisol, were significantly lower in the meditation group. This led the scientists to conclude, "Long-term deep meditation may have a beneficial effect on gut microbiota, enabling the body to maintain an optimal state of health."[12]

You do not have to be a Buddhist monk to improve your gut via meditation. Another study found that a basic nine-week training program to learn how to use spiritual tools such as meditation and prayer to elicit a relaxation response had a significant impact on participants' clinical symptoms of chronic gastrointestinal disorders such as irritable bowel syndrome (IBS) and inflammatory bowel disease (IBD), including Crohn's disease and ulcerative colitis, and even on the level of inflammation and the body's stress response.[13]

for at least fifteen minutes a day, learn a few yoga techniques to keep her body moving, and nourish her body with a diet consisting mostly of whole foods along with prebiotics and probiotics.

Beverly followed my recommendations. She also started tutoring children with special needs who attended the school affiliated with her church, which gave her purpose and a ready-made community. Within three months, her gut symptoms were under control, and she was on her way to recovery. She still missed her husband, of course, but along with her gut health, her anxiety and mental state improved dramatically. She was a true health hero!

I saw the same thing with my dad. Before he had his stroke, my father had been such an intelligent, creative, and busy man all his life. He loved what he did for work, and he found it hard to stop or even slow down. For him, retirement was not a relief but a stressor. So as he reached his seventies and retired, he began to lose his sense of purpose. And with that went much of his sense of community. Even though we have a tight-knit family, and he was always a very spiritual person, losing his work community was a big blow for him.

When my dad had his devastating stroke, many of the medical professionals he saw gave our family very little encouragement. Early in his course of treatment, Dad was transferred to in-hospital rehabilitation, and on his first visit the lead doctor told my sister and mother there was no hope for him. As you can imagine, this was a crushing blow. When I returned that evening after my hospital rounds, I was saddened to see the dejection on the faces of my family. The following day, I spoke to the attending physician and his colleagues and questioned their assessment after such a limited evaluation. I wanted our medical advocates to be just that: advocates for his care.

Despite the dire predictions, my family and I did not give up on Dad, and ultimately, we proved this doctor wrong. Although his purpose could no longer be new inventions, cooking delicious meals, or singing beautiful songs, we found ways to give Dad's life meaning, like setting a goal for each day, such as raising a spoon to his mouth or doing simple exercises even though he was wheelchair-bound. We built a community of family members, physical therapists, speech therapists, and other caregivers. When he had a success, even the smallest one, we celebrated that and prayed for continued progress, and it all gave Dad purpose. And we changed his diet, of course, making sure he had the nutrition he needed to help him attain his goals.

We paid attention to all those modalities, and as the Five Pillars were rebuilt, my dad defied the doctor's prediction. Six months after his stroke, he was sitting up by himself, watching television, and eating. He was still an older man who had had a stroke and still suffered deficits, but some of his physical ability and a great deal of his cognitive ability were restored. It took patience, and this is another key: time. Very rarely does any sort of healing happen overnight. We live in a society where we want everything now—faster, easier—but recovery is incremental.

Remember, you can use the simple, evidence-based tools in this book on your own, even if you do not receive encouragement from your healthcare team. Keep in mind that the Five Pillars are not magic or a cure-all—just as gut issues are not the only cause of cognitive decline. But, as you shall see, they are certainly an integral factor.

SIMPLE AND EFFECTIVE SOLUTIONS

While gut health may not be the only factor influencing cognitive decline, it plays a large enough role to make a significant difference in outcomes. Every day we learn about new and fascinating ways that the science supports this. For example, when fecal matter from a mouse that has Parkinson's disease is transferred into the gut of a healthy mouse, the healthy mouse often begins showing a telltale sign of Parkinson's—decreased levels of dopamine, the "feel-good" brain chemical. The gut microbiota of the patient with Parkinson's typically produce smaller amounts of short-chain fatty acids, which, as you will see in Chapter 1, are important in protecting the brain.[14]

Worldwide, an estimated 20 percent of people suffer from poor brain health, and most never fully recover. These dismal rates are not for lack of trying. With the advent in the early 2000s of functional magnetic resonance imaging (fMRI), which measures brain activity, and other imaging techniques, our understanding of how the brain works has increased significantly. Still, in the ever-changing, super-specialized world of medicine, one specialist is not always aware of the latest advances in another specialty. A neurologist, for instance, may be familiar with the basics of gut microbiome research, whereas a gastroenterologist might be just peripherally aware of the latest advances in addressing the neurofibrillary tangles of Alzheimer's disease. As a gastroenterologist passionate about cognitive health,[*] I live in both worlds.

---

* Throughout this book, I use "cognitive health" and "brain health" as synonyms.

And in my medical practice, I prescribe simple but effective solutions to patients and watch how their gut health symptoms improve in tandem with cognitive symptoms.

Gut health issues are ubiquitous these days. In the United States alone, an estimated 60 to 70 million people suffer from some type of digestive disease, like chronic constipation, diverticular disease, gallstones, hemorrhoids, reflux, IBS, IBD, and more.[15] Some of these people have no signs or symptoms, appear healthy, and have no idea they have a bigger underlying problem. The majority (including my dad) experience some discomfort, but they do not have enough pain to warrant a visit to the doctor or hospital, even though they may feel that something is not quite right. Even those who go to the doctor do not necessarily receive a diagnosis or a treatment. Twenty years ago, the doctor would have prescribed antacids (providing temporary relief but not a cure) or told you to eat more fiber (still a good recommendation). Ten years ago, your doctor might have suggested a probiotic and sent you on your merry way. Nowadays, we know gut health treatment is not "one and done."

Until recently, identifying what ails the gut has been hit or miss and treatment a process of trial and error. Is it something in the diet? Toxins? Stress? Advances in diagnostic tools are quickly giving us specific answers, focusing on the problem so that we can target the solution.

We are learning, for example, that developing Alzheimer's is not preordained even if you are genetically predisposed to it. Despite your family history, suffering a stroke does not have to be your future. And Parkinson's can be avoided or minimized.

Aging does not have to mean cognitive decline. You do not need to feel like you are on a speeding train and must brace yourself for the inevitable crash. You can take charge of your health.

By becoming a health hero, you really *can* unlock the potential to heal your gut and save your brain.

CHAPTER ONE

WHAT HAPPENS IN THE GUT DOES NOT NECESSARILY STAY IN THE GUT

once read an article claiming that children who ate dirt were less likely to be obese than those who lived a more sanitized existence.[1] As a gastroenterologist, I have read a lot of interesting research about gut health, but the connection between dirt and obesity was news to me.

It turns out every gram of dirt has more than 1 billion bacterial cells—many of which are good for the gut, contributing to a balanced microbiome, the collection of bacteria and other microorganisms (microbes) that naturally live within the intestines to help us digest our food. This striking research linked obesity to what the study authors called an "obese microbiota," or an imbalance of gut bacteria that causes the body to take more calories from food than a "lean microbiota" would.[2] Even if two people are eating the same portions of the same foods every day, for instance, the person with the obese microbiota might gain weight while the person with the lean microbiota might lose weight. The researchers concluded that for some people, obesity has little or nothing to do with how much or how little they eat. For example, they may simply lack *Bacteroidetes*, a group of bacteria that can be found in soil.

My reason for sharing this story is not to suggest that you eat dirt to lose weight (which is not a good idea for several reasons, including that much of our soil is contaminated). The article, published back in 2006, was significant because it attracted a lot of attention and opened up a world of research regarding the gut microbiome. Although the role of microbes in digestion was understood, researchers wanted to know what other powers these bugs held. If the composition of the microbiome could make some of us obese, could it also cause other diseases? If so, would it be possible to cure an illness by targeting specific microbes in the gut?

Since that article was first written, we have come a long way. Over the last two decades, researchers have published more than 25,000 papers on the gut microbiome, connecting it to conditions as diverse as autism and heart disease—disorders that, on the surface, would seem to have no common denominator. New tools and technologies have made it possible to study the microbiome more closely, leading to major advances in our knowledge about the role the gut plays in not only our physical health but also our mood and behavior. And as we now know, gut health can affect brain health.

Take the story of Katherine, for instance. She began to suffer from brain fog and forgetfulness in her mid-fifties. She felt she was too young to be having these kinds of problems, especially as the episodes grew more extreme. She consulted with my colleague, Dr. Steven Masley, who, after ruling out menopause and major illnesses and disorders as causes of her symptoms, made a few simple suggestions: he suggested she stop eating refined flour and sugar and add antioxidant-rich berries, cherries, and leafy greens to her daily diet. Katherine followed his simple advice and was relieved and thrilled by how her mind cleared and her memory returned. And she is not alone—in my years of practice, I have seen how even minor changes to our diet can improve brain processing speed and how we age.

BRAIN-BOOSTING BLUEBERRIES

- Not only are blueberries delicious and packed with potent antioxidants that boost immunity and help fight chronic diseases, such as cancer, heart disease, and diabetes, and lower blood pressure, but they are also great for your brain.
- Blueberries are often referred to as "brain berries" because they seem to improve cognitive function and memory, help delay age-related cognitive decline, and protect against depression.[3]
- Older adults who consumed blueberry juice every day for twelve weeks improved their memory and cognitive ability.[4]
- This is likely because brain-boosting blueberries contain anthocyanins, potent antioxidants that have been linked to improved brain function.[5]

Linking the condition of our gut with that of the brain may seem illogical at first, but mounting evidence and many success stories like Katherine's suggest repeatedly that what happens in the gut does not always stay in the gut. Just as eating well can benefit us, I have observed that doing the opposite and cultivating an unhealthy gut can lead to the destruction of neurons—those normally well-protected brain cells that are so central to our thoughts and memories and to our ability to focus, learn effectively, and direct our limbs to move on command. More and

THE BASICS: WHAT HAPPENS TO THAT BITE OF FOOD?

- When we take a bite of food and chew it into smaller pieces, the enzymes in our saliva begin breaking down the starches and fats into nutrients we can more easily absorb.
- We swallow, and food travels to our stomach (which is a muscular organ), where it mixes with acids and enzymes—gastric juices from the liver and pancreas—that break down the proteins, carbohydrates, and fats into something called chyme.
- This chyme is pushed into the small intestine, where the nutrients from the digested food enter the bloodstream.
- Waste products are sent into the large intestine, where they mix with most of the bugs in the microbiome and eventually are eliminated.

more, I have seen how poor gut health can be associated with some of the most feared neurodegenerative conditions of our time, including stroke, Alzheimer's, and Parkinson's.

Why would evolution give the gut the power to prevent us from remembering where we left the car keys or to determine whether we can pick them up off a table? Scientists are still trying to determine the "why," but we do know that as the microbiome developed over many thousands of years, the connections between the gut and the brain were simultaneously established, leading to these cognitive functional associations. Further understanding of the link between the gut and the brain begins with understanding how integral the gut is to our overall health and survival—and how connected it is to the rest of the body.

IT TAKES GUTS TO SURVIVE

An essential part of our gut is the large intestine (often called the colon), a five-foot-long organ neatly coiled and packed into the lower abdominal cavity, just below the waist. This lengthy digestive organ might seem as if it is trying too hard to fit into its allotted space, but its design is intentional. The large intestine is responsible, among other things, for helping us digest our food by absorbing water, producing vitamins, and forming and eliminating waste (feces). Digestion takes time, and so requiring food to move slowly through a long, curved tube makes sense. It takes about six hours for food to reach the large intestine after you eat it. Even in healthy individuals it can take up to an additional thirty hours before the gut is finished with your meal.

The gastrointestinal tract is a pathway that begins with the mouth and works downward, moving nourishment from the throat to the esophagus, stomach, small intestine, large intestine, rectum, and finally the anus, where elements of food the body does not need or cannot absorb are eliminated.

Whenever we consume food, the gut's microbes are happy, as they are being fed, too. Our nourishment is their nourishment. Microbes eat what they can digest and leave much of the fats, proteins, and carbohydrates for us. They *metabolize* our food for us, turning it into forms we can use to fuel our bodies. They also break down or ferment indigestible substances such as fiber, which our bowels use to form feces to move waste out of the body.

As our microbes metabolize the food we eat, they also create a group of substances that are key to our health: *metabolites*. Metabolites are molecules that include short-chain fatty acids (SCFAs) such as butyrate and acetate, which help maintain gut barrier function. SCFAs are a subset of fatty acids produced by microbiota during the fermentation of partially digestible and nondigestible polysaccharides—carbohydrates like starch and cellulose, consisting of a number of sugar molecules bonded together.[6] SCFAs are especially good for the gut lining, helping to keep it strong and intact, kind of the way moisturizer keeps our skin supple. When we decide what to have for dinner, most of us do not consider the impact our food choices will have on metabolite production, but what we eat affects whether microbes and the gut can produce a sufficient number of metabolites to keep us healthy.

Without the right combination of good microbes, the body cannot optimally use the nutrients contained within our meal, and so our bodies do not have the needed energy to function. Indeed, it takes guts to survive.

MICROBES: EARTH'S FIRST COMMUNICATORS

The gut itself is more than just a place where microbes eat and feces form. It is an ecosystem of microbes, neurotransmitters, genes, metabolites (like SCFAs and amino acids), immune responses, and much more. These substances work to keep much of our body functioning optimally. They do so through a highly intelligent communication network with ancient origins that began with the microbiome.

Billions of years ago, microbes that lived in the oceans evolved to develop a communication system. Just as humans would later use a smile or a grimace as signals to communicate feelings and intent, the microbes learned to "talk" to one another via molecules.[7] When one microbe signaled another by producing a particular molecule, it had an effect: the recipient of the molecule—the receptor—changed its behavior. For example, the autoinducer-2 (AI-2 microbe) signal molecule appears to be universal and facilitates communication between bacteria. AI-2 helps these bacteria to activate certain genes through a mechanism known as quorum sensing.

Roughly 600 million years ago, some microbes took an evolutionary leap by finding their way into multicellular organisms that were beginning to take shape in the oceans. These organisms were little more than tiny digestive tracts. The microbes helped their multicellular host organism thrive by aiding digestion. The host provided a ready and constant source of nourishment for the ever-hungry microbes. As microbes populated these developing guts, they brought their communication system with them.

This early communication system evolved into what we now call the enteric nervous system (ENS), which is composed mostly of neurons—the same type of cells found in the brain, but in this case lining the digestive tract. The ENS's main job is to carry out the cellular communication that facilitates digestion. Its origins (remember, it first developed in an organism that did not have a brain) ensured that the ENS can do a lot on its own, without any help from the organism's brain. This independence has led many to refer to the ENS as the "second brain." In truth, it is the first, as the brain in our heads along with the rest of the central nervous system (CNS) evolved much later.

The gut microbiome and the ENS have since developed a highly sophisticated long-distance communication system, with cells in the gut able to instantly direct cellular activities elsewhere in the body, including the brain. Much of this communication takes place along a well-established route called the gut-brain axis.

THE GUT-BRAIN AXIS: YOUR PERSONAL FIBER-OPTIC CABLE

Like a fiber-optic cable that reaches across continents, under ocean floors, and through mountains to enable communication between two distant and distinct countries, the brain and the gut are neurologically and biochemically connected via millions of nerves, billions of neurons, and the trillions of microbes that populate the intestines. Known as the gut-brain axis, this communication network between the two organs is a bit lopsided, with the gut wielding more influence over the brain than the brain has over the gut.[8]

By linking the gut and the brain, the axis connects the nervous systems associated with each of these organs as well—the ENS and the CNS. Even though the ENS does more of the talking, this communication is constant and bidirectional, going both ways.

The "fiber-optic cable" is the vagus nerve. Stretching from the brain down to the intestines, the vagus is the body's longest cranial nerve, one of the twelve paired nerves in the back of the brain. As such, it helps to regulate a wide assortment of bodily functions, ranging from our ability to swallow to our blood pressure. It also shares some responsibilities with the gut—namely, digestion and immune system responses.[9]

The gut-brain axis sends messages via the vagus using chemical messengers—neurotransmitters—that originate in either the gut or the brain. Microbes in the gut, for instance, produce 90–95 percent of the body's serotonin, a neurotransmitter responsible for stabilizing mood, sleep patterns, and appetite—all activities believed to be controlled by the brain.[10]

Or are they?

By producing neurotransmitters such as serotonin, the microbiome can use the gut-brain axis to influence activities in the brain. If the gut produces too little serotonin, for instance, we tend to feel depressed, sleep poorly, and eat too much. The gut is *that* powerful.

Despite the distance between the gut and the brain, the two are intricately connected and, as noted, it is a two-way street: gut communicates with brain, and brain with gut. The connection is profound, and you have no doubt felt it yourself. When the brain senses danger, for instance, we feel it in our digestive tract—that sinking feeling in the gut. The anxiety we feel before a speech might manifest as what we call "butterflies in the stomach."

Partly because of this connection, we know that what happens in the gut does not necessarily stay in the gut. If the microbiome

BOOSTING COMMUNICATION VIA THE GUT-BRAIN AXIS

Recent studies have shown that noninvasive methods of vagus nerve stimulation can increase and enhance communication between the gut and brain. Transcutaneous auricular vagus nerve stimulation (taVNS) done via electrodes has shown promising therapeutic efficacy,[11] but there are other, more accessible ways to stimulate the vagus, like:

- Gentle self-massage from the ears to the abdomen and all the way to the feet.
- Deep-breathing exercises.
- Cold-water immersion.
- Yoga asanas, or poses, including child's pose, forward fold, and savasana (the last of which is breathing deeply and slowly while lying on your back with arms and legs stretched out).[12]

is somehow compromised, it is unable to optimally carry out its many functions. The signals it sends to the brain via the gut-brain axis may be muddled or incomplete, my research and experience show, but the body's built-in "fiber-optic cable" has no choice but to deliver them to the brain.

So, what can impair the microbiome? What distinguishes a healthy gut from an unhealthy gut?

THE MICROBIOME: A WORLD UNTO ITSELF

Composed of trillions of microorganisms, the microbiome that lives within your large intestine is a world unto itself. The number of microbes in your gut microbiome is so large that the microbes taken all together weigh an average of two to four pounds. There are more microbes in your gut than there are people on Earth. But like the planet, your microbiome is also diverse, housing microbes of many different types and species, including viruses, bacteria, fungi, and protozoa. Think about this: you are carrying a universe that includes trillions of microorganisms with you all the time. It gives poet Walt Whitman's famous line "I contain multitudes" a whole new meaning!

When we are healthy, the organisms living together are balanced. Not only do we need them balanced, but we need them all. This diversity is essential. Science is beginning to show that the diversity of the microbiome is associated with the prevention of obesity and chronic illnesses such as type 2 diabetes, heart disease, and neurodegenerative disorders.[13]

Many of the species within the gut existed in prehistoric times. In fact, the origins of two of three major taxonomic families of gut bacteria found in apes and humans can be traced to a common ancestor who lived more than 15 million years ago during the Miocene Period, when mammals such as bears, horses, and saber-tooth tigers first began to populate the earth.

The community of microbes currently residing in your gut developed through evolution and continues to do so. Their primary goal is and always has been quite basic: survival and reproduction. And your microbes are good at it. In the time it takes you to read this chapter, many of your microbes will have reproduced once or even twice, passing their genes to their offspring, which will also procreate.

As in any group of a trillion, there are bound to be a few troublemakers, and the microbiome is no exception. Some microbes are helpful, working to support the body. Others—say, a harmful strain of *E. coli* we ingest by eating undercooked meat—can wreak havoc in the gut. Both good microbes and bad microbes multiply, but if we have a critical mass of good microbes, they will crowd out the bad.

Our community of minuscule, ancient living organisms is constantly in flux. We start out assuming some of our birth mother's microbiome when we pass through the birth canal, which is covered in bacteria. This protects us as infants against some of the same viruses and bacteria Mom and most likely her forebears were protected against.[14] We are just beginning to learn what happens to the microbiome of babies born via C-section instead of the vaginal canal, where much of the microbiome is passed on from mother to child. While it is clear that the microbiomes of infants born via C-section have more microbes that were likely acquired in the hospital (and which may cause disease) as well as fewer essential strains, and children born via the vaginal canal have more diverse microbiomes, the long-term consequences of these differences—if any—are still unknown.

Consuming breast milk also contributes to our microbiome, and the microbiome continues to develop during childhood based on race, ethnicity, caregivers, and other social factors.[15] Throughout our lives, the microbiome changes and is dependent

GUT FEELINGS

When the gut is absorbing and creating nutrients and otherwise functioning as intended, we feel good. We have regular bowel movements and a lightness of being. We stop eating when we are full. We are generally energetic, and we tend to be happy, as the gut can affect mood via the neurochemicals it produces—including the "feel-good" neurotransmitter serotonin. And we are likely to be mentally "on our toes," thinking fast and with clarity.

If things are not going well in the gut, we might experience discomfort or even severe pain in the abdomen. Constipation, diarrhea, bloating, fatigue, and even too much or too little appetite are signs that something may be wrong. Poor gut health can manifest as gut irritation or evolve into a disease—colitis, Crohn's disease, colon cancer, and diverticulitis, to name a few.

And do not forget about the brain! My research and experience have convinced me that depression and anxiety are among the mental health signs of an unbalanced gut.

on microbes contained in what we ingest (mainly food and drugs), the chemical toxins in our environment, any viruses or bacteria we are exposed to, and our stress levels, which increase the proliferation of unfavorable bacteria, crowding out beneficial species.

Different individuals' microbiomes include many of the same standard microorganisms, but each of us carries a unique combination and balance of microbes. In a sense, your microbiome has its own signature. The diversity also changes throughout our life span. Newborns, toddlers, and aging adults tend to have the least diversity and also are the most susceptible to certain illnesses, like diabetes and obesity.

Our microbiome is constantly changing, partly because of our behavior and our environment. As you will soon learn, although we cannot change the structure of our gut, we can change the composition of the microbiome for better or worse.

THE GASTROINTESTINAL BARRIER: THE BODY'S BORDER CONTROL

The gut is the destination for many substances that come our way through the food and drugs we ingest. The mucosal lining of the gut, known as the gastrointestinal (GI) barrier, is essential to filtering the barrage of substances that can enter the gut. Think of it as a border control with the power to determine what can enter the rest of your body—that is, what can pass through the barrier and enter the bloodstream—and what must stay in the gut or exit the body.

To make these decisions, to distinguish the good from the bad, the GI barrier relies on the intelligence of the ENS. It "knows" what will cause problems. Some of the bad actors include harmful bacteria, viruses, and other foreign substances such as the pesticide residue on the apple we just ate. Ultimately, the destiny of most of these unwanted molecules is to exit the body as waste as quickly as possible. If you have ever had the stomach flu, you know what I am talking about.

Although the GI barrier is a fortress, it also needs to be permeable enough to allow nutrients (for example, digested fats, proteins, and carbohydrates) to pass into the bloodstream, which carries them throughout the body for our tissues, organs, and muscles to use or store for energy, growth, and repair.

The GI barrier's permeability, however, is also its greatest vulnerability. If the GI barrier weakens, it may become too "loose," enabling larger "bad actor" molecules to escape from the gut into the bloodstream. Our body's major line of defense has lost some of its guards.

Another way to think of it is to imagine using cheesecloth to filter a vegetable broth you just made. If the cloth's fibers are intact, the broth flows freely through the cloth into the jar below, while the whole spices and carrot and onion remnants, for instance, collect on the cloth and you can easily discard them. If the fibers of the cheesecloth are too loose, however, some of these bits and pieces are allowed to pass through and cloud your broth.

The GI barrier was designed for strength and resilience—it is too important to our health and well-being to be easily damaged. But it relies on a constant supply of "good" gut microbes to maintain it and keep it strong. If these microbes are somehow missing or out of balance, the microbiome is unable to produce its normal supply and variety of metabolites—those substances, such as SCFAs, that are so essential to keeping the GI barrier strong and intact.

CHANGE YOUR MICROBIOME, CHANGE YOUR HEALTH

Like the rest of the body, the microbiome works best when in homeostasis—when all is balanced and functioning as intended. But because anything that goes into the body can affect the microbiome, either disturbing or enhancing it, paying attention to what we ingest or are exposed to is important. Nutrition, drugs, and toxins are some of the more obvious means of affecting microbiome composition. But do not forget about the other four pillars: movement, purpose, community, and spirituality.[16]

For now, let's use nutrition as an example. Diets that include too many highly acidic foods (think coffee and soda), foods high in saturated fat (such as ribeye steak), high-sugar foods (candy and many prepackaged foods and sauces), or too many high-protein foods (for example, if someone eats so much meat and seafood that they don't get enough other nutrients) also tend to be low in prebiotics and probiotics—two elements necessary for good gastrointestinal health—and devoid of postbiotics, which are equally essential.

Prebiotics are often the nondigestible parts of a food—namely, the fiber found in whole foods such as fruit and whole grains. We cannot digest fiber, but the gut uses it to form feces and help move waste products, including "bad" bacteria, out of the intestine. Low-fiber diets, as most of us have been told, are associated with constipation. Without fiber, the gut does not have what it needs to keep us "regular."

When fiber is present, microbes in the gut known as *probiotics* ferment the fiber to break it down so that it can pass through the final portion of the intestinal tract. (Remember, we can also ingest probiotics in the form of supplements or fermented foods or drinks like yogurt, kefir, sauerkraut, kimchi, kombucha, tempeh, cottage cheese, and even wine). As probiotics break down fiber, they secrete specialty chemicals known collectively as *postbiotics.*

While many people are familiar with probiotics, postbiotics are not a common topic of conversation. But the more we learn about the microbiome, the more we have come to understand the significant role postbiotics play in supporting the immune system, preventing cancer, stabilizing blood sugar, improving skin, treating allergies, and alleviating symptoms of irritable bowel syndrome.

An example of a postbiotic is butyrate, the short-chain fatty acid metabolite I talked about earlier. Butyrate is the preferred source of energy for the GI barrier. This is one reason every nutritionist will tell you to eat a diet high in fiber. When we eat enough fiber, probiotics can ferment it to create butyrate and other metabolites. When butyrate is present in abundance, the GI barrier is able to maintain its integrity. Butyrate is also a known anti-inflammatory.

When the pre-, pro-, and postbiotic symphony of microbial events is allowed to take place—supported by a healthy diet high in fiber, for instance—the gut microbiome is in balance. Our microbes get to eat, thrive, reproduce, and do their jobs. Constantly bombard the gut with processed foods low in nutrients and high in unnatural ingredients, mixed in with frequent antibiotics, and the gut microbiome has to adjust. It will digest pretty much whatever we give it, but when the symphony of microbial events is missing something—say, an essential nutrient or fiber—it is as if the horn section left the stage too early. With a shortage of fiber (prebiotics), for example, the probiotics have little to nothing to ferment and production of postbiotics wanes. Our symphony orchestra is not playing in rhythm or is out of tune.

The same is true if we give the microbiome too much of something the body does not need, such as high fructose corn syrup. Even too much of a good thing such as protein can be harmful, altering the chemistry of the microbiome so that it becomes unbalanced and less diverse.

But there is more. An unbalanced diet sets off a chain reaction. In addition to not producing the friendly bacteria the body needs for optimal health, the microbiome begins to produce harmful substances. Two of these are lipopolysaccharides (LPS) and trimethylamine N-oxide (TMAO). These substances are known mediators of inflammation—one of the main drivers of poor brain health and of cognitive decline. It's important to know what these mediators of inflammation are, so that we can prevent inflammation from occurring. One important way to do this is by focusing on the GI system, because as my colleague and friend Dr. Tom O'Bryan put it, "The biggest trigger for inflammation is what is at the end of your fork!"

CHRONIC INFLAMMATION: AN IMMUNE RESPONSE GONE WRONG

Chronic inflammation is a buzzword in the medical field because it has been associated with almost every chronic illness known to humankind, including cardiovascular disease, cancer, arthritis, type 2 diabetes, stroke, Parkinson's, Alzheimer's and other dementias, and much, much more. As opposed to acute inflammation—the result of things like bronchitis or an infected cut—which is a temporary immune response, chronic inflammation lingers for weeks at a time or longer. It usually begins as a normal acute inflammatory response that has gone awry. Think of it as a soldier that is still on the battlefield fighting long after the war has ended.

But what does inflammation in the gut have to do with heart disease? And how is it possible that an inflamed gut can affect our cognition—our ability to think clearly? It all starts with an innocent immune response.

The immune system is not centrally located. Immune cells and other immune mechanisms are located throughout the body—and, in fact, 70 percent of the body's immune system is in the gut. Immune cells rely on a highly developed communication system to keep each other informed—the same (albeit more advanced) communication system the ancient microbes first developed billions of years ago. When an invader is present, molecules called cytokines signal inflammatory cells (including white blood cells) to trap and isolate an unwanted substance by creating inflammation.

If you have ever sprained a joint, broken a bone, or suffered a hematoma (bad bruise), you have witnessed the immune system firsthand. The area around the injury swells as blood filled with inflammatory cells rushes to the area to trap "bad" bacteria and begin the healing process. A fever is also an inflammatory response. To defend the body against infection, the immune system raises the body's temperature to help kill off the pathogen. So even though it can be temporarily uncomfortable, an acute inflammatory immune response protects the body. Problems arise when the inflammatory response lingers and becomes chronic.

There are several reasons inflammation may turn from acute to chronic. Defective cells, autoimmune disorders such as lupus and rheumatoid arthritis (in which the immune system mistakes healthy tissue for an enemy invader), and long-term exposure to chemical irritants are some examples.

Physicians have often associated chronic inflammation in the gut itself with gut disorders such as Crohn's disease and celiac disease. But as we know, what happens in the gut does not necessarily stay in the gut. An unhealthy gut microbiome—triggered, say, by an unhealthy diet or a food allergy—can lead to physiological changes that activate the immune system inappropriately, causing an inflammatory cascade that can linger and lead to disease states that surface outside the gut.

For instance, a diet low in fiber means reduced production of butyrate and other helpful SCFAs. Without these SCFAs, we see increased amounts of the harmful substances the microbiome produces, such as LPS and TMAO—those mediators of inflammation. Low-fiber diets have been associated with bowel cancer, diverticulitis, and other inflammatory diseases.

The immune system is an immensely powerful thing. It is your CIA, FBI, state police, and army combined, keeping a close eye on "enemy" activities. However, it can be indiscriminate, setting off an inflammatory response whenever it senses a threat. The presence of excessive amounts of LPS, for example, simulates an infection. The body sees LPS, senses an attacking marauder, and unleashes its inflammatory response.

Over time, the effect on the microbiome becomes increasingly apparent in the form of uncomfortable and even painful symptoms: gas, bloating, diarrhea, constipation, cramping, and more. These symptoms often reflect a condition called gut dysbiosis—imbalance in the gut. The gut microbiome has become imbalanced—not enough good microbes and too many bad microbes. This imbalance is likely accompanied by less diversity as well.

Dysbiosis has bigger consequences, as it can lead to a condition called leaky gut syndrome, whereby LPS and other particles meant to stay in the gut are allowed to escape into the bloodstream.

LEAKY GUT SYNDROME

If you know much of anything about the Byzantine Empire, you have likely heard of the fall of its capital, Constantinople (present-day Istanbul), and the empire itself. It happened back in 1453, at a time when cannons, swords, arrows, and axes made up most of the weaponry—brutal, but nothing along the lines of today's capabilities.

Constantinople's fall was not surprising, as the city had been weakened over the centuries by naval forces and numerous sieges. What was surprising was the fall of the city's wall. For more than a thousand years, a wall four miles long, sixteen feet thick, and up to forty feet high had protected the city from invaders by land. It even withstood heavy cannon fire. That is, until it met Mehmed II, leader of the Ottoman Empire.

During a fifty-five-day-long siege, Mehmed's forces repeatedly bombed the wall with cannonballs. The constant stress of the cannonball blasts eventually weakened the structure enough

COMMON SYMPTOMS OF LEAKY GUT SYNDROME

- Acne
- Brain fog
- Chronic diarrhea or constipation
- Fatigue
- Fibromyalgia
- Gas and bloating
- Headaches
- Intense cravings, especially for sugar and carbs
- Joint pain and arthritis
- Memory trouble
- Mood disorders
- Pain
- Rashes, eczema, rosacea
- Thyroid conditions

that it fell, permitting Ottoman forces to enter this most protected of cities.

I offer this story not as a lesson in history but as a metaphor for how what happens in the gut can affect the brain. A gut lining constantly besieged by inflammation eventually wears thin and loosens, allowing "forces" meant to stay in the gut to enter the bloodstream. This is increased intestinal permeability, commonly known as leaky gut syndrome.

The leak does not have to be a gaping hole. A simple loosening that creates a tiny crevice is enough to allow "bad" substances to pass through the barrier—a molecule of LPS, for instance. The body is prepared for occasional events in which unwanted substances get through the barrier. When this happens, the immune system swoops in and attacks the unwanted substance so that it either can't enter the bloodstream or is prevented from making it too far.

If the GI barrier continues to suffer from inflammation, however, the lining, like the wall of Constantinople, continues to weaken, allowing more and more unwanted substances to pass through this once highly secure border and into the bloodstream.

Now we have a continuous feedback loop. Inflammation initially caused by diet or toxins loosens the GI barrier, permitting unwanted substances into the bloodstream. In addition, the postbiotic (produced by the microbiome) butyrate is not available in sufficient quantities to feed and repair the gut lining. The immune response, led by cytokines signaling inflammatory cells to stop the invader, creates more inflammation in the bloodstream. The compromised blood eventually makes its way up to the brain, where it meets another formidable defense—the blood-brain barrier (BBB).

The BBB is a cellular wall designed to protect the brain from potentially damaging toxins, pathogens, and inflammation circulating in the bloodstream. But it too can weaken when repeatedly damaged by inflammation, exposing our most precious of organs to not only toxins but also rogue immune responses that destroy brain cells and other tissue. This is how inflammation can affect brain health, leading to cognitive decline and even degenerative disorders such as Alzheimer's.

NEURODEGENERATION AND COGNITIVE DECLINE

Neurodegeneration is the term for deterioration of neurons, specialized cells designed to deliver key messages within the brain and throughout the rest of the nervous system. Via electrical impulses and chemical signals, neurons instruct our hand to pick up a glass of water when we are thirsty. They are the reason we can feel the warmth of the sun—and appreciate it. Neurons lead to actions, thoughts, and emotions. Throughout life, neurons connect with one another to create neuronal pathways in the brain—pathways that help us remember people, places, and things. Neurons form our memories.

Neurons are nothing to take for granted, as their supply is limited. Not long after we are born, the body stops producing most neurons. Although we can create new neuronal pathways—memorize a math formula or remember a new way to drive to work, for example—when neurons die off, the body typically will not regenerate them.

When we talk about neurodegeneration, we are not just talking about people becoming lost in the parking lot. The effects can be subtle or pronounced. Another way to talk about it is to think in terms of poor brain health or cognitive decline. The brain is not functioning optimally. This can involve forgetting where the car keys are, taking longer than usual to get through a recipe (brain fog), or a reduced ability to perform usual tasks, such as using a lawn mower.

With neurodegeneration, neurons are not functioning properly, perhaps because they are not getting necessary nutrients as the result of a disruption in blood flow (as is the case with stroke) or because inflammation is breaking them down. Either way, the results are damaging and usually irreparable. Although it may not be reversible, neurodegeneration is preventable. The more we learn about the gut, inflammation, and the brain, the clearer it becomes that gut health strongly influences brain health. Healing the gut, then, can truly save the mind.

GUT ATTACK

The microbiome is a remarkable structure living and thriving within our bodies. The immune system is probably the most complex system in the human body. And the gut, thanks to the neural cells in the GI tract, is second only to the brain in complexity. This synchrony among all these organs and systems is incredible, yet it is overlooked because we tend not to think about it. If the brain gets disordered, if the synchrony is not present, there is chaos—and once that occurs, it is often too late to reverse the damage. Doctors and their patients pay attention to heart health and lung health but tend not to notice when GI health is diminished. We test for and are concerned about a heart attack or a brain attack (stroke), but we do not think of the gut and its state of health. We don't address a gut attack when health is attacked and in disarray. It is time to change that.

CHAPTER TWO

GUT HEALTH: A STATE OF DIS-EASE

In the United States about one in five people suffers from a digestive disease like acid reflux, stomach ulcer, IBS, Crohn's disease, or even lactose intolerance.[1] A few of these folks have acute symptoms like vomiting and bleeding that bring them to my office or even to the emergency room. Some of them have symptoms such as bloating, constipation, or diarrhea that they may feel are not serious enough to call for a visit to the doctor. Many associate their discomfort with certain food types or ingredients—like dairy or gluten—and self-diagnose (or mis-diagnose) themselves as being intolerant. Others have no idea what is bothering them, and a considerable number may have no symptoms whatsoever.

My dad, for instance, had a history of gastric ulcer and knew that certain spicy and acidic foods were off-limits. He avoided anything that aggravated his ulcer. When he didn't, he experienced occasional discomfort, but not enough to make him think twice about the situation. He was like many of us whose health may have been declining so gradually that we are either unaware of it or think it is a natural progression of aging. Dad ate what he thought was a balanced diet. What he did not do was make a concerted effort to make gut health a priority. A lot of the people in his community, including doctors and family members, could have paid more attention, but many of them were not aware of how to optimize gut health.

Looking back at my dad's history, and having treated many more patients since his diagnosis, I now know he experienced subtle changes that could have alerted us to his declining brain health. A brilliant man, my father, Dr. Uma Nandi, gradually became a little more mortal. Complex calculations that had once been simple began to give him pause. His memory was not quite as sharp as it used to be. In hindsight, one example was especially poignant. He was driving and became lost and could not find his way back home. When he eventually returned, his charm and wit enabled him to explain this incident away as a transient lapse, and by doing so he diverted his doctors from suspecting that his brain health was deteriorating. Perhaps an intervention could have made a difference later, but hindsight, as we all know, is 20/20.

If we are to use the digestive tract to preserve brain health and prevent its decline, we need to make a practice of improving gut health and pay attention to even these "little" things. I would argue gut health needs to be our number-one wellness goal, but before we can find the solutions, we need to understand the problems, because when we are able to spot the warning signs and take preventive action, there is so much we can do to treat dis-ease before it becomes acute disease, or maybe even before it occurs at all. Think about this in terms of my dad's case after his stroke: if you can bring someone who is essentially incoherent and has been written off by his doctors to a point where they are able to eat by themselves and be attuned to the people and world around them, imagine what you could do proactively—addressing the health potential before there is a crisis.

HOW HEALTHY OR UNHEALTHY IS MY GUT MICROBIOME?

- Most of the time, we know intuitively whether our microbiome is off: our digestion is not what it usually is. For example, we may be experiencing flatulence or constipation, or perhaps foods we have always eaten no longer agree with us.
- If this persists, it is worth checking in with your doctor. One thing they might do is suggest a stool sample test. This will analyze the bacteria, fungi, and other microorganisms in your digestive tract and tell you if there is an imbalance.
- Depending on the type of testing, what your doctor learns might give you some insight into chronic conditions such as Crohn's disease, ulcerative colitis, or celiac disease.
- Home tests are readily available, but I recommend doing them in conjunction with a physician or other expert who understands not only the data but your health history as well.

RAISING A RED FLAG IN OUR BRAIN

Remember how I said what happens in the gut does not stay in the gut?

When you experience poor gut health in its extreme, you may suffer from bloating, abdominal pain, discomfort, nausea, vomiting, and changes in the way your bowels move. Those are common clinical signs. However, before these show up you may notice more subtle indicators, like having difficulty tolerating or enjoying the kinds of foods that you normally did. You might even experience episodes of "brain fog" or a feeling of mental ineptitude following your meals or at other times when, although you are satiated and well rested, you are not able to function well.

These relatively common and (at least on the surface) "normal" conditions can mask bigger troubles in the gut and/or develop into larger and more systemic issues, such as another autoimmune disease like lupus and rheumatoid arthritis, as well as celiac disease, type 1 diabetes, and psoriasis. These occur when the immune system mistakenly attacks parts of the body, in effect hurting itself to protect itself.

In other words, autoimmune diseases and their related symptoms could be signs of poor GI health, which then can contribute to, worsen, or even lead to poor brain health. It is important to watch for subtle signs:

- Distractibility when you have always been able to read and quickly assimilate information.

- Forgetfulness to a degree that feels inappropriate or uncomfortable.
- Irritability, emotional outbursts, confusion, and depression.
- Memory loss or a sudden change in mental energy.
- Not being able to follow conversations.
- Suddenly having trouble with basic computation when you have always been good at math.
- Trouble with recollection even when you are well rested.

People do not always see these as central nervous system or brain health issues, especially at first, but when you lose some of your cognitive ability and there is an abrupt shift in how you control your anger, stress, focus, or emotions, this may well be an effect of a disruption along the gut-brain axis.

As soon as we notice any of these symptoms, it is important to pay attention to what is going on with our gut because what we do not know (or what we ignore) can kill us. Many people think that unless there is an absolute dumpster fire in their abdomen, they are okay. That is not the case. Even if you are not bloated, uncomfortable, constipated, or having diarrhea every day, you still may have inadequate gut health. You may have mild or intermittent symptoms and blame them on over-indulgence—the chili you ate for dinner or that extra scoop of ice cream. In retrospect, I know my dad's gut health likely was not great. That is why it is important to pay attention—our gut can act as a barometer forecasting harsh weather in our body and especially our brain.

MECHANISMS AND FACTORS OF POOR GUT HEALTH

The healthy gut is one that is functioning properly. It is doing what it is supposed to, which is to absorb nutrients and not cause symptoms. But beyond that, at a microscopic level it is helping your entire system be more robust. To me, the gut is the center of all health. It is the place where you can either preserve health or not, because the integrity of the GI system—that protective barrier between the gut and the blood, which impacts the rest of your body—must be very stable and not compromised, or else you are going to have problems. Yet we do so many things to destabilize it.

Numerous factors play a role in this and in how certain conditions like irritable bowel syndrome and reflux often worsen as we age. Genetics is one such factor—a family history of Crohn's disease or celiac disease, for example. We might not have much control over these (although, as you will see in the next chapter, we are not powerless), but we can impact our gut health by paying attention to the things we put into our mouths and the lifestyle choices we make, especially within the context of the Five Pillars that I discussed in the introduction.

CARBOHYDRATES AND SUGARS

Many of my patients have gut problems because their guts are in a state of dis-ease, plagued by a diet high in unhealthy fats and refined sugars and low in the nutrients that produce neuroprotective substances such as short-chain fatty acids. It is important that we make thoughtful choices at every meal. A nutrient-rich breakfast with fruits and oatmeal, or a donut? Salad or fries? Or what about the last kids' birthday party you attended? There is a good chance the menu included pizza, cake, ice cream, and soda. But if you think about it, the foods we celebrate with are no cause for celebration—pizza is an atomic weapon launched straight to the gut, and the unfavorable carbohydrates are problematic even for the healthiest person.

Let's start with carbohydrates.

Carbohydrates are key components in nutrition and are one of the three basic compounds in food (the other two are protein and fat) that provide us with energy. The main forms of carbohydrates are sugar, fiber, and starch. Despite popular media describing carbs in very unfavorable terms, not *all* carbs are "bad." In fact, most healthy adults' diet should be composed of about 50 percent carbohydrates. The type of carbs you eat is critical, and a key factor in gut problems is "bad" carbs.

However, what is a "good" and "bad" carb? "Good" carbs are typically plant-based foods, with their fiber intact. Veggies, fruits, nuts, and seeds along with whole grains (like whole wheat, brown rice, oats, barley, quinoa, and millet) are high-fiber sources of "good" carbs. "Bad" carbs include sugary treats and foods made from white flour, such as baked goods, and refined grains, such as white bread and white rice. These foods lose most of their fiber during processing, giving you "bad" carbohydrates.

What make some carbs "good" and others "bad"?

Our bodies digest and absorb fibrous "good" carbs slowly, allowing them to deliver energy in a gradual, sustained way, with gentle effects on our blood sugar levels. It is a healthy process and how our bodies were designed to work. On the other hand, "bad" carbs, which skip the fiber, are digested and absorbed quickly. This makes you hungry again soon after eating, which leads to overeating, weight gain, and opting for easy choices like fast food. It also makes you feel lousy (there is that gut-brain connection again) and can increase the risk of developing a variety of diseases. This can be the result of a sudden and unhealthy spike in blood sugar (glucose) levels, soon followed by a crash.

Foods are ranked according to something called the glycemic index, which indicates how fast that food affects your blood sugar level. Foods that contain absolutely no carbohydrates have a glycemic index value of 0, and pure glucose (sugar) has a value of 100. Glycemic load is another indicator that can tell you how the food you eat affects your blood sugar, and it is calculated by multiplying the food's glycemic index by the total amount of carbs contained in the quantity of that food you eat at any given time.

Healthier carbohydrates have a lower glycemic index. Green vegetables have a low glycemic index, as do legumes, such as lentils, beans, and soybeans. Most whole grains and fruits have moderately low to moderate glycemic loads, so they can be a significant source of carbs in a healthy diet. Starchy foods such as potatoes can have a moderately high glycemic index. These carbs should be an occasional treat rather than a daily staple.

Where the problems start is at the high end of the glycemic index. White bread, pastries, and packaged snack foods—pretty much anything made with refined grains—along with sodas, energy drinks, most juices, and most processed foods have the highest glycemic loads. These should be avoided as much as possible. Not only do these foods have little to no nutritional value, but they are often high in calories, supplying energy in the short term, but this energy is not sustained. Worst of all, they supply a feast for "bad" bacteria in our gut, throwing our microbiome out of balance and effectively destroying or diminishing the good bacteria we rely on.

NOT ALL FATS ARE CREATED EQUAL

Just as there are "good" and "bad" carbs, so too are there "good" and "bad" fats, which pretty much divide up as unsaturated and saturated fats. Not only are saturated fats bad for your waistline

BAD CARBS IN DISGUISE

At first glance, some packaged foods that might seem healthy (or at least neutral) are not.

- "Low fat" does not necessarily mean "low sugar."
- "Sugar free" or "diet" is different from "fat free."
- "Light" products and artificial sweeteners are no better. According to research conducted on animals, sugar substitutes have a negative impact on the microbiome. When mice were given artificial sweeteners, their blood sugar levels rose, and they had trouble using the insulin their bodies produced.[2]
- Foods that we might not think of as high on the glycemic index often have "hidden" sugars, so read the labels on flavored yogurt, pasta sauce, salad dressing, and ketchup carefully.

and your heart, but when it comes to the gut-brain axis, they also decrease gut health and, as a consequence, make optimal brain health unachievable.

Unsaturated fats tend to be liquid at room temperature. This category of fats can be broken down into monounsaturated and polyunsaturated fats. Monounsaturated fats are usually plant-based and can be found in foods like olive and peanut oils, pumpkin seeds and sesame seeds, almonds and cashews, and avocados. These are all good for us in moderation, not only because they help lower bad cholesterol and raise good cholesterol as well as improve the control of blood sugar levels, but also because they support a more balanced microbiome, helping optimize gut health and subsequently brain health.

Polyunsaturated fats consumed in moderation can be good for us as well, mainly because they contain omega-6 and omega-3 fatty acids. These fats can be found in oily fish like salmon, anchovies, mackerel, herring, sardines, and tuna, as well as soybeans and walnuts. They lower the levels of triglycerides ("bad" fats) in the blood and can decrease our risk of heart disease.[3]

Thus, they help our gut in many of the same ways monounsaturated fats do.

Those are the good or pretty good fats. The bad ones are saturated and trans fats. Saturated fats are usually solid at room temperature. Meats like beef, lamb, pork, and poultry, especially with skin, have elevated levels of saturated fats. So do dairy products like butter, cream, and any whole-milk product. These bad fats tend to raise levels of low-density lipoprotein ("bad" cholesterol) in the blood. Too much LDL in the bloodstream increases our risk of heart disease.

Trans fats might be the sneakiest of the bad fats. They are made from plant oils that have been chemically altered (partially hydrogenated) to become a solid fat. They can be found in foods like margarine, nondairy creamer, microwave popcorn, and many frozen meals. Although trans fats are inexpensive and have a long shelf life, the US Food and Drug Administration (FDA) has deemed these artificially created fats unsafe, so avoid them whenever possible.[4]

Studies have already shown that industrially produced trans fats are associated with increased inflammatory markers when they replace other nutrients in the diet.[5] As you will see later in this book, there is emerging evidence that high intake of saturated fats and high cholesterol levels can also be linked to a greater risk of Alzheimer's and other types of dementia.

ABOUT GMOS

According to the FDA, genetically modified organisms (GMOs) are foods that have had their DNA altered through genetic engineering. They were developed to save money and grow crops more effectively, helping farmers increase yield, prevent crop loss, and control weeds. But does the good outweigh the bad? I'd say no. Not only do GMOs negatively affect biodiversity on the planet, but eating genetically altered foods may also have a negative and even toxic effect on our liver, pancreas, kidneys, and reproductive system, as well as our immune system.[6]

FOOD OR POISON?

Of course, fat and carbohydrates are not the only things affecting our gut. What is used to produce even the healthiest foods—such as kale, brown rice, and broccoli—can be harmful, damaging our overall health and GI systems. Chemical fertilizers and synthetic pesticides added to fruits and vegetables, as well as often unsafe antibiotics, medications, growth hormones, and unhealthy food given to livestock that is slaughtered for meat, all, to one degree or another, put poison on our plates, ultimately going from our bellies to our brains.

The most efficient way to avoid this is to eat organic. The word *organic* describes how foods are grown and processed. Organic fruits and vegetables are grown using natural fertilizers, and weeds and insects are controlled by tilling, weeding, bug traps, and natural pesticides instead of toxic chemicals. Organic livestock is fed organic non-GMO feed, and diseases are prevented with natural methods like a varied diet, clean living space, and safer antibiotics and medications.

In my practice, I have found that patients who eat organic foods reduce their risk for certain diseases as well as obesity. Many of my patients were happy to see their GI and other symptoms lessen or disappear when they focused on maintaining an organic diet. Here are some of the reasons this happens:

- Organic foods contain fewer pesticides. When these chemicals are used on conventional produce and the soil in which it is grown, they remain in the food you eat—they are in the cells, so no amount of washing can remove them. Essentially, then, this means that when we do not eat organic foods we are consuming low doses of bug and weed killers.

- Organic foods do not contain preservatives to give them a longer shelf life, so you can be more confident that what you are buying is fresh.
- Organic produce, dairy products, and meats are richer in many nutrients, such as omega-3 fatty acids, than conventionally produced foods.
- Organic produce is often more nutritious and has a higher vitamin content than conventional produce.
- Organic produce is free from GMOs, which have been linked to diabetes, cancer, and neurological defects.[7]

Another danger on our dinner plate is highly processed foods. These can be defined as foods made from ingredients extracted or refined from whole foods, and many of them have a high glycemic load. Diets high in soft drinks, lunch meats, TV dinners, canned soups, chips, and cookies are low in dietary fiber, micronutrients, and phytochemicals and high in bad fats, sugars, and sodium.[8] They tend to contain additives, especially chemicals intended to make the product appear more attractive, taste sweeter, or stay fresher longer. Researchers have found a connection between highly processed foods and adverse health outcomes such as allergic and autoimmune disorders, some types of cancer, cardiovascular disease, and metabolic disorders including type 2 diabetes and obesity.[9] Furthermore, because highly processed foods tend to taste good as a result of their high fat, sugar, and salt content, we end up eating too much of them. So, protect your gut, brain,

AFFORDABLE ORGANIC AND NON-GMO FOODS

We are often told to buy organic and avoid chemicals in our food, but sometimes this can become an expensive undertaking. Here are a few suggestions that can help:

- Shop sales and wholesale markets. If you find produce you like at a competitive price, buy extra and freeze it.
- Frozen fruits and vegetables (not prepared meals) tend to be less expensive and have no significant difference in nutrition compared to fresh. They also tend to have a higher concentration of nutrients than fresh foods stored in a refrigerator for many days.[10]
- Join a community-supported agriculture (CSA) program at a local farm that can provide organic foods for the entire growing season. Many of these offer sliding payment scales and even accept Supplemental Nutrition Assistance Program (SNAP) payments. And again, if you have extra produce, freeze it.
- Grow your own! Even a few vegetables in pots on a sunny windowsill can supplement your healthy food intake.
- If you cannot buy everything organic, avoid the Environmental Working Group's "Dirty Dozen" foods (when nonorganic), those with the highest amounts of pesticide residues:[11]
    1. Apples
    2. Blueberries

3. Cherries

4. Grapes

5. Green beans

6. Greens

7. Nectarines

8. Peaches

9. Pears

10. Peppers

11. Spinach

12. Strawberries

- Substitute the "Dirty Dozen" with the "Clean Fifteen" foods—those that tend to have the lowest amounts of pesticide residues—when you can:[12]

1. Asparagus

2. Avocados

3. Cabbage

4. Carrots

5. Frozen peas

6. Honeydew melon

7. Kiwis

8. Mangoes

9. Mushrooms

10. Onions

11. Papayas

12. Pineapple

13. Sweet corn

14. Sweet potatoes

15. Watermelon

and health in general by doing your best to avoid things like cake mixes, instant noodles, many ready-made meals, and prepared frozen foods.[13] In other words, frozen berries and spinach are great, but TV dinners and pizza—not so much.

BEYOND FOOD: ANTIBIOTICS AND OTHER MEDICATIONS

It is not just the food we eat. Often when we take prescribed medications, we believe we are making a healthy choice, but this is not always the case,[14] especially when it comes to antibiotics. Our microbiome is like a miniature ecosystem, and as we've seen, we want to preserve good bacteria and not introduce bad bacteria. However, since antibiotics kill *both* good and bad bacteria, the microbiome can be disrupted for up to six months after antibiotic treatment. So if your doctor recommends a prescription antibiotic, ask if this is the only and best choice.

Do not get me wrong: antibiotics have many benefits and have saved innumerable lives from potentially fatal infections like sepsis, strep, and bacterial pneumonia. I prescribe them when required, but it is essential to understand how to use them wisely and take our gut health into consideration. When we take antibiotics, it's important to up our intake of fiber, prebiotics and probiotics, and fermented foods.

In 2018 researchers gave an intense regimen of powerful antibiotics to young, healthy men for four days, and over this time almost all their gut bacteria were wiped out. The participants were followed over the next six months, and most of the subjects' bacteria populations went back to the levels measured

HYPERPALATABLE FOODS: BUYER BEWARE!

Many large corporations tend to be more concerned with their profit than with our health, especially when it comes to hyperpalatable foods (HPFs). These are processed foods like candy, chips, cookies, french fries, and cheeseburgers, which combine high levels of sugar, sodium, fat, and/or carbohydrates to activate the brain's reward system, stimulating excessive eating and actually fostering addiction. A study published in 2022 revealed that many leading food companies which disproportionately developed and marketed HPFs are owned by US tobacco companies, which had decades of experience misleading and manipulating consumers.[15]

before the study. However, nine distinct species of good bacteria were still missing.[16] This loss of diversity, if not rebalanced, could have long-term effects not just in the gut but throughout the body, including the brain.

THE FIVE PILLARS THAT AFFECT GUT HEALTH

Looking at gut health within the context of the Five Pillars, we are reminded that although nutrition plays a key role in our health, it is only one part of the equation. Not only is improving and sustaining gut and brain health about eating nutritious foods and having a sense of purpose, but it is also about adequate movement, without which we are at risk for many related diseases. You have probably heard people talk about sitting being the new smoking. That is because if we live a sedentary life, we are at about the same risk of having cardiovascular disease, strokes, or other fatal diseases as someone who is a smoker. Likewise, lack of movement leads to fatigue, joint pain, muscle aches, and general malaise. When it comes to the physiology of our GI tract, if we do not exercise, we encourage lack of diversity in the microbiome and thus poor GI health.[17]

SIGNS YOUR MICROBIOME MAY BE UNHEALTHY OR OUT OF BALANCE

- You have digestive problems like bloating, indigestion, diarrhea, nausea, or IBS.
- You do not eat a healthy diet.
- You are addicted to processed foods and sugar.
- You are overweight or obese and have difficulty losing weight.
- You have a poor immune system and have frequent respiratory issues, infections, and gastrointestinal problems.
- You are experiencing inflammatory health conditions (anything from allergies to heart disease and others).
- You have poor memory, anxiety, depression, or other mood disturbances. Remember, your gut is nicknamed your "second brain" for a reason.

Even community and spirituality are factors here. Research has shown repeatedly that inattention to these two pillars leads to stress. One fascinating example of this is the "Roseto effect," a term coined in 1961 to account for the unusually low rate of myocardial infarction (heart attack) in the Italian American community of Roseto, Pennsylvania. It is the basis upon which many following studies were created, including one done over a fifty-year period finding that members of this tight-knit and cohesive community lived healthier lives and experienced less stress.[18] But you do not have to be Italian American or live in Pennsylvania. Other studies like ones done by the Beckman Institute have shown that close friendships likewise reduce stress.[19]

Health heroes understand that reducing stress is key when it comes to gut health. It turns out that when we are less worried, anxious, or jittery we release less cortisol into our bloodstream; cortisol decreases inflammation, regulates blood pressure, lowers blood sugar, helps us rest, and makes it easier to bounce back after being upset or frightened. Chronic stress has other negative impacts. When we are stressed, we are more likely to binge-eat, especially highly processed or unhealthy foods. Additionally, stress hormones and the ensuing inflammation reshape the microbiome's composition, bringing us full circle, since "bad" gut bacteria may also exacerbate our stress response.[20]

DRAWING CONCLUSIONS

My dad's eating habits, like the habits of many other folks who experience a decrease in brain health, may have led to his brain's decline. He ate what he thought was a balanced diet, but what he did not do was make a concerted effort to make gut health a priority. In the years before his stroke, Dad would occasionally suffer from an upset stomach with some bloating and discomfort. It was transient and lasted for two or three days, but I now know that his GI tract was giving us some clues. This is where I think an intervention would have been useful. Had I said, "Hey, let's try to follow an even more plant-based diet and eat foods that can heal your intestinal tract," we might have seen another outcome.

What happened with my dad is what occurs in many doctor-patient relationships—both parties react only to severe symptoms. We do not see the warning signs. It is like we are on the *Titanic* and do not realize there is an iceberg ahead until it is too late to change course.

Although I wish I could have done something differently in my dad's case, we did not have the amount of data and evidence about the gut-brain connection that we do now. Sir William Osler, often described as the father of modern medicine, once said, "To study the phenomena of disease without books is to sail an uncharted sea, while to study books without patients is not to go to sea at all."[21] That is why in this book I am sharing with you the maps I wish I'd had back then.

CHAPTER THREE

HOW TO CHANGE YOUR GUT HEALTH

Despite all the things that can go wrong with our gut and all the ways we can damage our GI tract, there are a lot of ways we can help things go right as well as actions we can take to heal or improve the GI system. Remember my story about the benefits of children eating dirt? Every time we enjoy a meal—be it french fries and a hamburger, or kale and black-eyed peas—we potentially change our microbiome. How we make that change is up to us, but for healthy change to occur, we must *want* to do it.

Here's an example. My kids have a Nintendo Switch. To date, I have never had to remind them to charge it. Why? Because they have an important goal: to play with it. Folding their clothes, however, is an entirely different story, because neatly organized, wrinkle-free T-shirts don't seem to have the same level of priority for most eight- and ten-year-old children. They do not always care enough to make this a daily practice. The same thing is true for adults—incorporating anything into our daily regimen requires commitment and change.

Change, as most of us know, can be hard to sustain. But when a new habit has a purpose that we value—such as charging a treasured videogame player or eating food that supports the health of our body and brain—it's much easier. The best way to make something a habit is to have a goal that is important to you, and few goals in life are more important than saving our brain.

HOW TO MAKE GUT HEALTH A PRIORITY

I know my breakfast and lunch routines very well, because I am conscious of the types of foods I want to put in my body to achieve the results I desire. My dinners have a bit more variability and I do have an occasional restaurant meal, but in general I am extremely conscientious about what I eat. This comes from my quest for great health, which stemmed from my health challenges as a young boy, when I suffered from rheumatic fever, and I established good habits as a young man and physician. Seeing my patients' plight when they didn't pursue a healthy food plan and how their gut health suffered as a consequence was a great motivator.

I endorse the importance of great gut health in helping treat diseases of the GI tract, the brain, the immune system, and even the heart. Using my own experiences, I help my patients understand the critical importance of gut health in achieving true wellness. This is because although there are endless food options available to us, many of them are not at all compatible with a healthy gut. It is a daily challenge to make the correct choices to help your gut have a fighting chance. These choices are sometimes not easy to make and may require discipline and purpose. When the pursuit of excellent health is our primary goal, we can take steps to reach it. Deciding that this pursuit is our mission is a process, and taking the first step can begin to shift our behaviors. And solidifying this behavior—making it habitual—is the key.

Take Sam, for example. He suffers from Crohn's disease. He has been my patient for nearly a decade, during which I have counseled him on the importance of gut health through diet and purposeful living. It took him a while, but when he finally made it a practice to improve his eating habits, his life changed. Gut health is now a critical element of his plan to achieve remission from this dreadful disease. He has become a wonderful cook, creating beautiful and flavorful meals with whole foods and spices. Many of his dishes use turmeric and cumin, which are beneficial for the gut-brain axis. The results have been nothing short of spectacular.

MAKE IT A HABIT! FOUR TIPS TO IMPROVE GUT HEALTH

1. Do not eat out more than once a week.
2. Try to avoid processed foods and limit them to no more than 25 percent of your meals.
3. Consume organic, non-GMO foods as often as possible.
4. Eat with someone—dinners with family and friends help build the pillar of community.

STOP BEING SO SAD

There is a reason why the typical diet of a US citizen is called the Standard American Diet, SAD for short. Consuming primarily calorie-dense and nutrient-poor foods and beverages means eating a lot of "bad" fats and carbohydrates, not to mention large amounts of additives and pesticides, with little room for beneficial foods. When it comes to changing gut health, we all need to try to switch to a primarily plant-based way of eating. Even a minor change will immediately impact your gut health, so do your best to eat more:

- Vegetables, particularly leafy green and cruciferous ones.
- Alliums, like garlic and onions.
- Spices.
- Fermented foods.
- Berries.

As you shift toward a way of eating that heals your gut and saves your brain, apply the wisdom of author Michael Pollan, who famously said, "Eat food. Not too much. Mostly plants." In other words, eat *whole* foods, not processed or packaged ones; eat to *nourish* yourself, not to alleviate stress or boredom; and, most importantly, eat as much *plant-based food* as possible. Myriad studies have found that vegetarian diets benefit the gut microbiome due to their high fiber content. Some vegetables (like avocados) contain "good" fats, and no vegetable contains a "bad" fat. Research has also shown that plant-based foods are generally higher in the nutrients that increase the levels of beneficial bacteria in the gut while decreasing harmful strains of bacteria, not to mention packed with vitamins and minerals.[1]

Let's take a closer look.

Leafy greens. Leafy green vegetables offer nutrients like folate, vitamin C, vitamin K, and vitamin A and are tasty sources of fiber. Examples include cabbage, lettuce, and kale. Several studies have shown that these foods contain a "good" carb called sulfoquinovose,[2] which supports the growth of healthy gut bacteria. Thus, leafy greens help to build a healthy microbiome.

Cruciferous vegetables. Cruciferous vegetables like broccoli, Brussels sprouts, radishes, kale, bok choy, and cauliflower can be eaten raw or cooked. Either way they are incredibly nutritious, supplying protein, good carbohydrates, and vitamins (especially vitamin A, vitamin C, and folic acid) and minerals including iron, calcium, selenium, copper, manganese, and zinc. For example, 1 cup of cauliflower has 3 grams of fiber, which is 10 percent of what you need each day to feed the healthy bacteria in your gut, optimize colon function, and reduce inflammation, all things that promote digestive health.

Radishes, on the other hand, supply 1 gram of fiber per cup, but their leaves are especially beneficial. A promising study found that radish juice may help prevent and even alleviate gastric ulcers by protecting gastric tissue and strengthening the mucosal barrier. This is essential because the mucosal barrier protects the stomach and intestines against unfriendly microorganisms and damaging toxins that may cause ulcers and inflammation.[3]

Allium vegetables. If you ask me, everything tastes better with garlic, so add a little more whenever you are preparing savory foods. A study in *Food Science and Human Wellness* showed that garlic supports the proliferation of "good" gut bacteria (*Bifidobacteria,* for example) and prevents harmful bacteria from growing. Garlic is rich in inulin, a type of nondigestible carbohydrate that acts as food for the favorable bacteria in your digestive system. Raw garlic is best for gut health, as it loses its prebiotic benefits the more you cook the garlic.[4]

Like garlic, onions of all colors (white, yellow, red, green) improve the flavor of almost every dish. Not only are they reliable sources of vitamin C, vitamin B6, potassium, and folate, but they are packed with antioxidants, which help protect cells in your body against damage from free radicals and fight disease. Onions are one of the richest sources of flavonoids (including quercetin, a natural pigment found in fruits and vegetables), phytochemicals with powerful anti-inflammatory properties, and can help heal a leaky gut.[5] Onions also have considerable amounts of prebiotics and fiber.

Spices. Equally important are spices. Take ginger, for instance. We may think of it as something commonly used to flavor cookies, but it is delicious in savory foods as well and has many medicinal properties. Ginger can help relieve nausea, vomiting, and other stomach-related symptoms. In a study published in the journal of *Food and Chemical Toxicology,* researchers found that ginger can increase our levels of prostaglandins, which are hormone-like substances.[6] Prostaglandins function to increase the ability of the gut lining to absorb more of the nutrients our bodies need. There are also compounds found in ginger called gingerols. These have been shown to have anti-inflammatory properties, which may be why this spice works so well on digestion problems.

Incorporating a variety of spices into your diet may improve digestion, metabolism, nausea, and overall gut health. However, if you add only one new spice to your diet, make it turmeric. I try to incorporate it into all my meals. It is a great anti-inflammatory agent and is gut-protective. More American grocery stores now stock fresh turmeric root. The dried ground variety can be used too, but check the best-by date and opt for organic whenever possible. Turmeric has antioxidant abilities that thwart inflammation, and it has been shown to boost brain health, increase memory, and lower the risk of heart disease by improving the function of our blood vessels.[7] Being anti-inflammatory, turmeric is a natural analgesic—it can fight acute pain as well as ease chronic pain, and it is much better for our gut than other anti-inflammatory meds called NSAIDs, such as ibuprofen, aspirin, or naproxen. Because turmeric is fat-soluble, eating it with a meal containing healthy fats makes it more effective. Better yet, add black pepper to your turmeric-rich dishes: the piperine in the black pepper makes turmeric 2,000 times more bioavailable (the degree to which a substance is available for biological activity or use by the body)![8]

Fermented foods. While you are making changes to heal your gut, be sure to add the fermented foods mentioned earlier and the pre-, pro-, and postbiotics they contain to your daily diet. Food that has undergone fermentation—where yeast or bacteria break down the sugars they contain—include:

- Cheeses that have been aged but not pasteurized or heated, including cheddar, Swiss, provolone, Gouda, Edam, and Gruyere.
- Cottage cheese.
- Honey (raw).
- Kefir.
- Kimchi.
- Kombucha.
- Sauerkraut.
- Tempeh.
- Yogurt.

Many of these are high in *Lactobacilli*, a probiotic that is good for your microbiome health. According to research, people who consume yogurt on a regular basis have lower levels of bacteria linked to inflammation and several chronic illnesses.[9] To reap the gut health benefits from yogurt and cottage cheese, be sure the label reads "contains live cultures" or "contains active cultures."

Berries. Fruit is always an excellent choice, and berries are the best. In my clinical experience, most berries help chronic inflammation and improve gut bacteria. Berries are among the healthiest foods available and are an excellent alternative to sugary snacks. Consume a few servings of berries every week and experiment with different varieties.

Eight of the top berries for gut health are:[10]

- Açai berries
- Bilberries

- Blueberries
- Cranberries
- Goji berries
- Grapes (yes, grapes are berries!)

"PLANT-BASED" DOES NOT ALWAYS MEAN "GOOD FOR YOU"

- Fast-food restaurants and grocery stores now offer all kinds of plant-based "meat" that includes healthy-sounding ingredients like peas, rice, mung bean protein, coconut oil, cocoa butter, potato starch, vinegar, and beet juice extract. But eat them in moderation; they are more like a treat than a healthy alternative.

- The amount of sodium and saturated fat in plant-based "meat" is often the same or more than regular meat products.

- Fast-food chains fry their alternative meat products the same way they do their regular meat products. Combined with a white-bread bun and a side of greasy fries, they may be plant-based, but they are certainly not good for your gut.

- Keep the focus on eating real, whole foods as often as possible. If your only choice is fast food, opt for salads, tacos without the tortillas, burrito bowls, or wraps and subs that are mostly vegetables.

- Raspberries
- Strawberries

EXERCISE AND GUT HEALTH

Returning to the Five Pillars, we know that movement can be almost as important as nutrition when it comes to making positive changes in our gut microbial composition, since our gut microbiota play a role in energy homeostasis and regulation. What exactly does exercise have to do with our microbiome?

Quite a lot, as it turns out. Studies have found that regular exercise increases species diversity in your microbiome and reverses gut imbalances related to obesity.[11] Regular exercise effectively changes your gut microbes. Recent research has shown that lifestyle changes that included several weeks of exercise resulted in an increase in participants' levels of butyrate, the metabolite that keeps our gut happy by reducing inflammation and producing energy.[12] Another benefit from regular exercise was more diverse gut microbiota, which often means better health. As we've seen, with a reduction of microbiota comes an increased risk of disorder-causing inflammation.[13]

Low-intensity exercise like cycling, walking, and yoga can reduce transient stool time—how long our feces stay in our colon—and the contact time between pathogens and the gastrointestinal mucus layer or GI barrier. As a result, researchers are finding that exercise can help reduce the risk of colon cancer, diverticulosis, and inflammatory bowel disease[14]—all good news for our gut.

MY FAVORITE EXERCISES FOR OUR GUT (AND BRAIN)

- Cardiovascular exercises like brisk walking or running
- Yoga
- Tai chi
- Biking
- Sit-ups or abdominal crunches
- Pelvic floor activators like Kegels

Scientists in Ireland have found that professional athletes have far more diverse microbiomes than their less-active peers. As expected, athletes and nonathletes differed significantly when it came to inflammatory and metabolic markers like blood glucose, triglycerides, HDL cholesterol, waist circumference, and blood pressure. More importantly, athletes had a higher diversity of gut microorganisms.[15]

Being active outdoors, for instance, has been shown to alter the microbiome in children by increasing levels of *Roseburia*—a bacterium thought to prevent inflammation in the intestines—and fecal serotonin levels, which can help prevent constipation. This type of movement not only enhanced the children's connection to nature and prevented inflammation but also improved behavior.[16]

YOU ARE NOT YOUR GENES

Something I find especially exciting is that even characteristics we believe are "hardwired," like genetics and aging, can be affected if we commit to changing our lifestyle and subsequently our gut. The cells in the gut, like all cells, have DNA, and the gut microbiome and many diseases can have an important inherited component. You can't change these, but it turns out that just because diseases like IBD or colon cancer run in your family, there are actions you can take that may shift the odds in your favor. What you eat can change your genes and transform your biology. This knowledge can be transformative, empowering everyone.

Since our genes play a role in everything, from the color of our eyes to our likelihood of developing certain diseases, it makes sense that they also play a role in our dietary requirements. DNA is a significant factor in figuring out what nutrients our bodies need and how we process the food we eat. For example, some people have genes that allow them to absorb certain nutrients from their food more efficiently. Others have traits that make them susceptible to specific food allergies or intolerances like lactose or wheat. By understanding our genetics, we can make better choices about the foods we eat and ensure that we get the nutrients we need. We can also use DNA testing to identify diet-related health risks and take steps to avoid them. In other words, DNA testing can help us tailor our diets to our individual needs and improve our overall health. For example, as healthy as it is, more kale may actually not be what *your* particular body needs; rather, you may benefit from eating more broccoli. Specific genes may allow us to undo the damage caused by unhealthy foods, and a new field of research into the connections between genetics and nutrition is changing the game.

Nutrigenomics is a new field of study focused on how nutrition affects your genome and can help turn genes on and off. This could mean a different life journey—an amazing, healthy, and happy one, possibly without falling prey to inherited diseases. Using nutrition to affect our genetic expression means we are no longer at the mercy of our DNA. Nutrition is a game changer when it comes to fighting and preventing disease. We are at the wheel, taking control, instead of being passive passengers in the pursuit of excellent health.

The idea behind nutrigenomics is that food can influence genes because our genes react differently to different nutrients. According to the *Journal of Microscopy and Ultrastructure* the primary principles of nutrigenomics are:

- Many diseases have diet as an important predisposing factor.
- Our genetic expression can be impacted by the foods that we consume.
- An individual's susceptibility to disease can be explained by genotypic variability.
- Genes can be affected by dietary factors. These genes can have a role in the development and progression of chronic diseases.[17]

For example, most of us are aware that some people are born lactose intolerant and others have no issues with cow's milk. Lactose intolerance in infants is often due to a mutation of the LCT gene, which provides information for making lactase, the enzyme used to digest lactose, a sugar found in milk. Many folks develop lactose intolerance as teenagers or adults because of gradually decreasing LCT gene activity, yet there are those in whom the gene continues to function well throughout their lives, and these people can drink milk happily.

Researchers have found that alterations in LCT gene activity are due to genetic changes not within the LCT gene itself but in nearby areas in the DNA molecule. In particular, single-nucleotide polymorphisms (SNPs), tiny variants in DNA in which one person's genome differs from another person's genome by just one base (one molecule), modulate the expression of the LCT gene. This is an example of what's called epigenetic modulation—how the way genes are expressed can change even if there's no change to the gene itself. Furthermore, our previous ideas that genes cannot be changed are no longer true. New techniques for altering gene expression in the body mean that the future is bright for patients with genes that lead to disease.[18]

Nutrigenomics is an emerging field. There is still a lot to learn, and more research and testing are needed. While nutrigenomics can help to prevent and treat many diseases, it is not a panacea for all health problems.

AGING AND CHANGE

Just like our genetic inheritance, most of us believe the associated ailments and limitations of age are inevitable. To a certain degree the changes associated with aging are indeed inevitable, but by understanding our gut-brain axis, we can take action to possibly slow the process and even, sometimes, reverse it.

Aging brings about a host of changes: our metabolism slows down, body composition shifts, and hormone levels change. We do not need as many calories to keep our body processes working well. As we get older, food can sit undigested in the stomach because the movement of food contents through the stomach slows. This can often cause digestive distress. Bloating and flatulence, IBS, small intestinal bacterial overgrowth, and decreased small intestinal movement can develop or worsen, too. This decline in the speed with which food passes through the GI tract, the onset of new diseases, changes in the diet, changes in a person's hunger and appetite, and changes in gut immune function can all contribute to gut health problems in our senior years.

Another important cause of dis-ease is the use of medications that slow GI motility—the contraction of the muscles that mix and propel the contents of our GI tract. These include medicines that so many in our mature population are prescribed (and perhaps overprescribed), like narcotic painkillers and anti-depressant medicines.

Our gut microbiota helps supply nutrients to our body and affects the immune system. After the introduction of solid foods in childhood, the gut microbiota gradually diversifies and tends to remain stable. However, this gut diversity tends to decline when we reach our senior years,[19] and there is an increase in certain types of bacteria that were previously not dominant, such as those that may be pro-inflammatory.

At the same time, there is a decrease in the number of *Bifidobacterium* strains present, leading to poor gut health and decreased immune health and increased inflammation. We know this is true because we have seen how microbial diversity in stools also decreases with age. As we get older, we may also experience an overabundance of coliform bacteria. These are

PROTECTING YOUR GUT MICROBIOTA AS YOU GROW OLDER

Aging brings different strains and limitations to our microbiome, so it is more important than ever to take care of it. Here are some things you can do:

- Ask your healthcare team if that new prescription (especially if it is an antibiotic) is necessary. Overuse of antibiotics can lead to decreased diversity and an imbalance of microbes *unless* your doctor intends to therapeutically manipulate your gut microbiota.
- Variety is the spice of life. As we age, we tend to eat a less diverse and even monotonous diet as a result of living alone, lack of motivation, or even depression, so try some of the recipes at the end of this book and mix it up.
- Add more probiotics to your diet. Food is best, but a supplement can be helpful as well.
- Do not skip your dental appointment. Problems with our teeth tend to make us favor soft foods and avoid ones like raw vegetables, fruits, and nuts that help our gut but require chewing.
- Keep moving. As we age, we tend to limit our physical activity because of mobility issues, fear of falling, or lack of incentive, but exercise has many benefits, including helping food move through our colon more efficiently and improving the composition of our gut microbiota.

rod-shaped microbes that can exert a negative influence on the rest of the microbial population. Given the vital role of the GI tract in the absorption of nutrients, these shifts in the microbiome can have a significant impact on the health of the elderly.

Research suggests that changing the gut bacteria may have a positive impact on the aging process. The implication is that protecting healthy gut microbes may help people live longer, healthier lives. As you age, make it a habit to start shopping for probiotic foods that will improve the number of good bacteria in your body. As I mentioned earlier, fermented foods are a reliable source of good bacteria to help in this quest.[20]

IF YOU DO ONLY ONE THING TO IMPROVE GUT HEALTH . . .

If you do only one thing to improve your gut health, that thing should be to find your kitchen!

Even if you cannot go vegan or give up the occasional cheeseburger, preparing your own food can radically change your gut and your brain. You may have read that the populations of countries like India and China historically have far less cognitive impairment and decline than is seen in the West. This may in part be due to using turmeric and cumin in cooking in these countries. Also, preparing foods at home and eating more whole foods is ingrained in these cultures—not because they have read about it in a book, but because this is their habit, their way of life, passed on from generation to generation. Also, many folks in these countries take a Five Pillars approach to meals, not solely in terms of the nutritional elements of their meals but also in the sense of community and even spirituality that accompanies their consumption of food.

Sadly, that is now changing, because fast-food restaurants with their menus of processed foods are everywhere around the world. The convenience and allure of prepared and hyperpalatable foods, easily accessible and often affordable, make the spread of these unhealthy options almost unavoidable. To preserve cognitive and gut health, we must counteract the effective marketing of these disease-causing foods.

Think about it. In the West, we can drive to a restaurant and have a plate of food put in front of us or even call a delivery service that will bring meals to our door. Not only do we not know what ingredients or additives are used, but in the most extreme case we do not even have to walk to the door—we can roll our desk chair down the hall to get it. I am being a little bit facetious, but not that much. Many of us do this every single day. The pursuit of convenience is shifting our habits in the wrong direction, eroding basic tools that help fight diseases.

That is why preparing your own food is so important. Not only does food taste better when you make it, but it changes your entire understanding and approach to eating. I involve my kids in this process. They think the food tastes even better when they help, and they enjoy the experience. The entire family—our little community at home—works together to solve problems creating our meals. When we then sit down together to enjoy the fruits of our labor, our tribe helps to solidify our health, one meal at a time, the health hero way.

CHAPTER FOUR

HOW GUT HEALTH CONTRIBUTES TO STROKE

A stroke is a vascular event—a "brain attack," if you will. When my father had his, it affected his entire left side, to the point of the initial paralysis of his left upper and lower extremities. You can compare a stroke to what happened when a tanker truck crashed under an Interstate 95 overpass in northeast Philadelphia in mid-2023 and the resulting fire caused the roadway to collapse; it was not a single lane that was affected but 160,000 regular commuters who usually took that route, causing ripple effects as far away as Maine and Florida. It was like that with my dad—so many connections were disrupted. To the untrained eye, it might have appeared that he just had difficulty with movement, but the stroke affected his cognition as well. The brain pathways through which information was processed were significantly altered, to the point that often he seemed unaware or unable to understand that he could no longer do certain things. He was also unable to express the difficulty he was having trying to process information and perform simple tasks.

Before he had his stroke, not a single doctor suggested Dad might be at risk for this devastating disease. No one recommended checking his microbiome; no one ever suggested he alter his diet or that he exercise or meditate to improve his gut and brain health. Nobody brought up the possibility that slowing down in retirement was not fun or a benefit for my dad—a brilliant polymer chemist who was used to being extremely social and accomplished, leading teams in cutting-edge research—but instead was a stressor for him. His physicians were not being remiss. Science had not yet made the connection between gut health and adverse neurological events. Even today, few doctors understand enough about gut health to make the connection between it and stroke.

There are so many things we attribute to aging, such as losing mental acuity or getting a little lost or confused for no reason, and perhaps we think there's nothing we can do about them. When something like that happens to a high-functioning professional, like my father, we tend to ignore it or write it off as an isolated or transient episode. But what if we approached such episodes as early warning signs (which, in my father's case, we missed)? I genuinely believe that if we had helped my dad make some gut health changes before he had his stroke, we might have had some impact on the severity of his stroke, and might even have prevented it. For example, if we had connected my father's GI symptoms to occasions when he transiently became confused, maybe we could have had an intervention and looked at how these events were connected with his gut and perhaps recommended changes in diet, supplements, and exercise. The problem was that I did not have the data about the gut-brain axis that I do now.[1]

In Chapter 2 we saw that research supports an association between risk conditions for stroke—hardened arteries, metabolic disease, obesity, inflammation—and an unbalanced microbiome. Even more fascinating, there seems to be a direct connection between an unhealthy microbiome and likelihood of stroke. According to a study that analyzed gut microbiomes, those with an unhealthy microbiome with less diversity were more likely

WHO IS AT RISK?

Risk factors for stroke include:[2]

- Lack of physical activity
- Smoking
- Being overweight or obese
- Heavy and/or binge drinking
- High blood pressure (hypertension)
- High cholesterol
- Obstructive sleep apnea
- Diabetes
- Heart disease
- Family history of stroke or heart attack
- Age over fifty-five
- Being African American
- Being male
- Using hormonal birth control or some hormone therapies

to be associated with stroke than those with a healthy microbiome.[3] Other studies support this, some finding that people with an unhealthy microbiome were still more likely to have a stroke even after adjusting for risk factors such as age, sex, race, and smoking.[4]

Some of the factors contributing to stroke risk are probably familiar, but there are surprising ones as well, and many of them are directly related to our gut. To understand these, we need to understand what a stroke is, who is at risk, and why.

WHAT IS A STROKE?

A stroke, or cerebrovascular accident, is also called a brain attack. More than 85 percent of stroke events are ischemic, which means they are caused by an artery clot or other blockage in a blood vessel leading to the brain. Subarachnoid hemorrhages are less common, the result of a sudden rupture of an artery in the area between the brain and the tissues that cover the brain. In either event, there is an interruption of the flow of blood, and thus oxygen, to cells in the brain. When these cells are deprived of oxygen, they become damaged or die, often causing lasting brain damage marked by changes to speech, learning, movement, and understanding. Patients experiencing stroke may have long-term disabilities, such as weakness or paralysis on one side of the body, and may even die.

A related condition is transient ischemic attack (TIA), sometimes called a mini-stroke. This is not actually a stroke, but an event that mimics stroke symptoms. This event happens when the brain stops working optimally for a brief period. It may only last for a couple of minutes. A TIA may be a sign that a major stroke is coming. In fact, one in three people who have a TIA will eventually have a stroke.[5] My mother was one of these folks who had a TIA and then suffered a stroke years later. When a patient experiences a TIA, there is a window of opportunity for intervention, when we can make a change to prevent further, more catastrophic events.

I have many patients who have experienced TIAs. They have received evaluations from their neurologist, internist, and even cardiologist, but hardly any have been counseled on their gut health. I often ask them how they have changed their food and lifestyle since the TIA. Typically, they have been instructed to adopt a low-fat diet and been informed that their cholesterol and lipid levels should be optimized. Rarely is a victim of a TIA asked about their understanding of their microbiome or gut health.

I feel that we have an opportunity, especially with patients who have experienced a TIA, to make proactive, preventative changes to ward off future catastrophes like the one my father experienced. The stroke robbed him of his golden years, time in which he could have been playing with his grandkids and sharing his brilliance with them. Understanding that we have this very real opportunity is critical to making changes for a healthy future for patients who have experienced TIAs and even some who have already had a stroke.

CAUSES OF A STROKE

The universally recognized causes of stroke include hardening of the arteries, obesity, and hypertension—persistently high blood

MAJOR SYMPTOMS OF A STROKE

When it comes to stroke, knowing the symptoms can be a matter of life and death, and time is of the essence. Every second your brain is without oxygen is exponentially more destructive. Here are some common symptoms:

- Sudden numbness or paralysis, most often on one side of the body, in the face, an arm, or a leg. One arm may fall limp, or a smile may become a droopy half smile.
- Trouble speaking—words become slurred, language is confused.
- Trouble understanding—having difficulty understanding speech and experiencing confusion.
- Sudden and severe headache without a reason; this may be accompanied by vomiting, dizziness, and disorientation.

pressure. Metabolic disease can be another factor. This is a cluster of conditions that occur together and include increased blood pressure, high blood sugar, excess body fat around the waist, and abnormal cholesterol, particularly triglyceride, levels. In combination, these factors increase your risk not only of stroke but also of heart disease and type 2 diabetes.[6]

Emerging research appears to be showing that each of these conditions—hardening of the arteries, obesity, and hypertension—can be independently linked to dysbiosis, or imbalance in the gut. When the gut microbiome does not have enough

- Trouble seeing through one or both eyes; blurred or blacked-out vision; seeing double.
- Trouble walking; loss of balance or coordination; sudden dizziness; uneven gait.

For unclear reasons, women experiencing stroke tend not to have as many of those typical symptoms. Often, they have more generalized symptoms or unusual symptoms. Less generally, symptoms that tend to appear more often in women include:

- Fatigue or weakness
- Nausea or vomiting
- Loss of consciousness
- Sudden hiccups
- Sudden shortness of breath

good microbes and has too many bad microbes, this imbalance is likely accompanied by less microbiome diversity as well. In other words, there may be too many harmful gut bacteria and/or not enough beneficial gut bacteria. Over time, the effect of dysbiosis on the microbiome may become increasingly apparent in the form of uncomfortable and even painful symptoms, such as gas, bloating, diarrhea, constipation, cramping, and more.

It is important to understand that dysbiosis may have bigger consequences. As we saw in Chapter 1, it can lead to leaky gut syndrome (increased intestinal permeability), whereby LPS and

IF YOU SEE SOMEONE HAVING A STROKE, FOLLOW THE "FAST" METHOD

- **F**ace: Ask the person to smile and check if you notice a facial droop on one side.
- **A**rms: Ask them to raise both arms and check if one drifts downward.
- **S**peech: Ask them to say a simple sentence and check for slurred speech, garbled words, or confusion.
- **T**ime: If you notice any sign of a stroke, even a minor one, call 911 immediately.

Do not hesitate or wait to see if symptoms go away. If it is a stroke, the patient needs immediate medical attention. The sooner help comes, the higher the chances of survival and recovery. Do not drive anyone who may be having a stroke, and do not drive yourself if you think you may be having a stroke. An ambulance is faster, and the EMS staff is trained to provide appropriate treatment until you reach the emergency room.

Call 911 even if symptoms disappear. It may be a TIA, which may last for only a few minutes, but could be a warning sign that a major stroke is on its way.

Strokes have various symptoms, and some of these may be similar to the symptoms of other conditions, such as multiple sclerosis, seizures, or even migraines. Strokes are a serious, life-threatening condition. Do not wait and try to figure it out yourself. If it is indeed a stroke, immediate help is crucial.

other potential toxins meant to stay in the gut are allowed to escape into the bloodstream. There they can cause inflammation and lead to disease in many parts of the body.

SURPRISING FACTORS CONTRIBUTING TO STROKE (THAT YOUR DOCTOR MIGHT NOT MENTION)

Nutrition

We know by now that what we eat affects our microbiome, but there is a direct correlation between nutrition and stroke as well. Many recent studies have indicated that people who eat too much of certain foods increase their risk of stroke.[7] Basically, the SAD so common in the West is killing us. The more we neglect eating foods high in fiber, and fruits and vegetables rich in vitamins and other nutrients, the more likely we are to have a stroke. In fact, healthy food choices such as those found in the Mediterranean diet (see Chapter 7) can decrease stroke risk by at least 40 percent in high-risk patients.[8]

The biggest culprits, according to recent studies, are saturated fats, processed foods (especially refined grains), and salt. Meals that consistently feature the triad of red meat, refined grains, and sweet desserts cook up the perfect recipe for a health disaster.

Bad fats. Saturated fat consumption can be correlated with stroke mortality for ischemic stroke.[9] We know that an abundance of saturated fat in the diet contributes to increased inflammation in the gut and decreased microbial diversity, leading to poor gut health.[10] In addition, in animal and human experiments, diets higher in saturated fat have been shown to lead to an increase in harmful gut bacteria and decreased beneficial gut bacteria. And because gut health has been shown to be associated with vascular health, reducing our intake of saturated fat helps our gut and subsequently our overall health.

Salt. Even a sustained daily salt intake of little more than a teaspoon (5 grams) per day was associated with a 23 percent greater risk of stroke. This is likely because sodium elevates blood pressure and causes fibrosis (scarring or thickening of the tissue) in the heart, kidneys, and arteries. We now know that high-salt diets change the composition of the gut bacteria and also affect the short-chain fatty acids they produce. Both gut bacteria and SCFAs may affect blood pressure and consequently the risk of stroke. Changing our dietary patterns to decrease salt intake to no more than 2000 mg per day is helpful in improving gut health and modulating the risk of stroke.[11]

Bad carbohydrates. Bad carbs tend to have a high glycemic index, and include not just cookies and white bread but also sugary sodas and anything with added sugar (like ketchup). Eating too many "bad" carbs can lead to a worsening of diseases such as diabetes, one of the metabolic disorders associated with stroke. Processed carbohydrates also decrease gut microbial diversity and can diminish gut health as well.[12]

Sleep

The foods most of us eat every day are not the only surprising contributors to stroke risk. According to the Centers for Disease

Control and Prevention (CDC), a third of adults in the United States do not get enough sleep. I have a challenging schedule and often struggle to get adequate sleep on a regular basis, but I have made it a priority. Unfortunately, my father also had a tough time getting the sleep he needed. Little did he know the impact this had on his life. Any overworked parent or young adult studying for exams can tell you how difficult it is to get some quality rest, but what you might not know is that studies have connected a bad night's sleep to an increased risk for heart attack *and* stroke. A 2018 study found that sleep disorders, especially sleep apnea, are common in those who are also at risk for stroke. As Michael Grandner, director of the Sleep and Health Research Program at the University of Arizona College of Medicine in Tucson, put it, "It's like with diet, every cell in the body benefits from food in some way. . . . Sleep is similar in that way. The whole body [benefits]."[13]

So many of us work hard—much of the time out of necessity—and in our culture it is often a source of pride, accomplishment, and even status. But habitually working long hours could put your health at risk. A study published in 2019 showed that continually working ten hours or more per day could increase your risk of a stroke. And we're not just talking about working a ten-hour day every day. The risk of stroke increases by almost 30 percent after working ten-hour days only fifty days in a year—about one day of overtime per week. So if you have been doing this for years, your stroke risk has increased by 45 percent.[14] Sadly, that is not where the bad news ends. The greatest stroke risk correlates with being over the age of fifty-five, but the risk is even higher if you are *under* the age of fifty and overworked.

When we don't get enough sleep, we find another surprising side effect: inflammation. Sleep deprivation can increase inflammatory cells and factors in the body. This can result in worsening health throughout our bodies. Inflammation is a characteristic of many diseases, and increased amounts of it in the body can lead to disease as well, which brings us back to the gut.

INFLAMMATION

Many patients are not aware of the importance of inflammation in disease states, even those of the cardiovascular system. A plaque may form in an artery, but the added presence of inflammatory cells can result in a series of reactions that cause blockage of the blood vessel. If this happens in the coronary arteries, a heart attack (myocardial infarction) can result.

Inflammation can be a product of poor gut health. With lack of diversity in the gut microbiome, unfavorable bacteria can dominate, producing substances that increase gut inflammation. With an increase in, say, LPS, systemic inflammation can occur, causing or worsening many diseases such as diabetes, autoimmune disease, and even stroke.

Research presented at the European Stroke Organization Conference 2022 showed that the state of our gut microbiome can affect the risk of stroke and post-stroke neurological outcomes.[15] Fecal samples of stroke patients have shown that increased *Fusobacterium, Lactobacillus,* and *Acidaminococcus* species in the microbiome are associated with poor stroke recovery.

With such unfavorable bacteria, an abnormal immune response begins and can result in runaway inflammation in the gut, influencing other organs in the body. From heart attacks to brain attacks, the body pays the price. An imbalance in the bacteria can result in increased clot formation—unfavorable bacteria can produce metabolites such as TMAO, which increases platelet hyperreactivity, and LPS, which can activate platelets to begin the clotting process.[16] An unhealthy microbiome may also contribute to stroke in the opposite way, by impairing the body's ability to clot blood. These are just more reasons it is critical to maintain excellent gut health and good microbiome diversity.

MICROBIOME RESEARCH AND STROKE RECOVERY

Scientists at the West Virginia University School of Medicine might have discovered a link between stroke patients' gut health and how they recover from a stroke. Their research focused on communication between the brain and the gut along the gut-brain axis. Although other research has explored the effects stroke has on the microbiome, how long these effects lingered was unknown, and the WVU researchers found some remarkable things.[17]

Looking at how the gut influences the brain and vice versa, Allison Brichacek, a graduate student in the university's immunology and microbial pathogenesis program and a member of associate professor of neuroscience Candice Brown's research team at the West Virginia University School of Medicine, compared microbiomes in animals that suffered an induced stroke to microbiomes in those that did not. The microbiomes were reviewed on the third, fourteenth, and twenty-eighth days following the stroke. The researchers also looked with a microscope at the intestinal tissue. The aim was to see if there was a connection between the stroke and the microbiome.[18]

At the fourteen- and twenty-eight-day points, *Bifidobacteri-aceae* was less prominent in animals who had had a stroke. These bacteria are found in many yogurts and in a number of probiotic supplements, and they are almost universally recognized as supporters of digestive health. Interestingly, presence of this bacteria might also be related to improved outcomes in stroke patients.

The researchers also found that at fourteen days, the ratio of *Firmicutes* bacteria to *Bacteroidetes* bacteria was six times greater in the patients who had experienced stroke, suggesting an increased ratio of bad gut bugs to good ones in these stroke patients. This is particularly notable, as high *Firmicutes*-to-*Bacteroidetes* ratios are linked to inflammation, diabetes, and obesity.[19]

The study further found that stroke can cause detectable intestinal abnormalities—intestinal tissues that appeared normal in the healthy animals appeared "scrambled" a month after the stroke in the post-stroke models. "There's disorganization here,"

FIRMICUTES AND *BACTEROIDETES*

More than 90 percent of our gut microbiota community consists of two groups of bacteria: *Firmicutes* species and *Bacteroidetes* species.[20] *Firmicutes* species are typically beneficial, anti-inflammatory bacteria, and *Bacteroidetes* species are typically "bad" and pro-inflammatory.

explained Brichacek. "There's also less space between the villi [projections from membranes, like those in the inner lining of the small intestine] to allow nutrients to move around."[21]

With disruption of the intestinal wall, increased inflammation can persist. Nutrient absorption, vital for health and stroke recovery, can become impaired. The healing that is so critical in recovery from a stroke can thus be hindered by compromised gut health.

As noted earlier, there is a two-way conversation going on: gut bacteria affect brain function, and the brain affects gut function. Some gut bacteria influence brain function through the production of short-chain fatty acids. As noted earlier, SCFAs help decrease inflammation and preserve gut health, and they directly affect the brain by helping to maintain the blood-brain barrier and by supporting the growth and preservation of brain cells. SCFAs are critical parts of the brain-gut connection.

Understanding this connection and its importance helps us realize that improving gut health may help prevent cognitive decline in stroke patients. Also, if we could lower the *Firmicutes*-to-*Bacteroidetes* ratio in stroke patients, it could help in many other ways, such as assisting with weight loss, decreasing diabetes risk, and even reducing the risk for further strokes.[22]

OUR "SECOND BRAIN"

The same team from the West Virginia University School of Medicine wanted to learn more about how breaches in the intestinal barrier (the mucous layer and epithelial cells) affect the central nervous system. Avoiding breaches is vital for the proper function of the enteric nervous system, which, as we've seen, is called the "second brain." Studying dysfunction in the gut-brain axis after a stroke may show us the way toward potential treatment and even prevention strategies for stroke.[23]

Of most interest to the researchers is how distress in the gut-brain axis—such as cytokine release, changes in the blood-brain barrier, altered microbiota, and leaky gut—can lead to the migration of inflammatory and immune cells from the gut to the brain. After a stroke, the blood-brain barrier changes, allowing inflammatory and immune cells to get into the brain. A study focusing on the exact molecular mechanisms involved in the changes to the gut-brain axis in post-stroke patients would be very helpful.

"People don't appreciate the gut. It controls much more than digestion," says Dr. Candice Brown, who is also a faculty member at the Rockefeller Neuroscience Institute. "Our results suggest that stroke targets both brains—the brain in our head and the brain in our gut."[24]

This research made me wonder: if we knew at the time my father had his stroke what we know now, could we have altered the ratio of bacteria in his gut? Might that have made his last years more pleasurable and not filled with frustration and struggle? How can health heroes change the brain in our gut to protect the one in our head?

CHAPTER FIVE

CHANGING THE COURSE OF STROKE

Treating stroke has traditionally been extremely difficult. Care is expensive, costing upward of $40,000 for the initial hospital stay alone. Approaching stroke prevention and recovery from the lens of gut health could be a game-changer.

Bill came to my office in the fall, complaining of changes in his bowel habits. He had suffered a stroke in early spring, which led to weakness of his extremities. At first glance, his treatment seemed to be comprehensive. He saw his neurologist regularly and received therapy from his physiatrist (a specialist in physical medicine and rehabilitation). He had vascular tests and an ultrasound of his heart (an echocardiogram). He was placed on blood thinners. However, there was no mention of his gut health or its role in the stroke. This is not uncommon, as the connection is not understood by many practitioners who treat stroke, but Bill wanted to be a health hero, so we set out to change that.

Stroke can result when a blood vessel is blocked with a blood clot forming at a vessel plaque, causing lack of circulation to that part of the brain. So it stands to reason that addressing the functioning of your vasculature (improving the efficiency of blood vessels) can help prevent a stroke. While traditional rehabilitation methods used for stroke should still be used, my novel therapeutic strategy focuses on the pathogenesis—the origin and development of the disease. And that includes examining the gut microbiome.

We can change the gut microbiome by employing several techniques:

- Using probiotics, beneficial bacteria, may help.
- Using prebiotics, which feed the healthy bacteria in your microbiome.
- Using whole and fermented foods that are favorable to the development of beneficial bacteria, thereby reducing the production of harmful gut metabolites.

These approaches also reduce inflammation and the risk of atherosclerosis (hardening of the arteries) and, beyond reducing the risk of stroke, can help control diabetes, improve insulin resistance, and reduce blood pressure.

USING PROBIOTICS

Probiotics can be a game-changer in altering your microbiome. The trillions of bugs in your intestine help multiple processes in your body. Optimizing the bugs in your gut is of paramount importance, not only for gut health but because it also helps decrease inflammation throughout your body. Supplements are an effective way to add probiotics to your diet and alter the level of favorable bacteria, especially at the beginning. Ultimately we should aim to do this with diet.

Once the probiotics are in your gut, they need to eat too. Giving them the right foods—called prebiotics—is critical to an optimal microbiome. Prebiotics are nondigestible nutrients—typically high-fiber foods—that enhance and encourage the growth or activity of beneficial bacteria in the gut. They essentially fulfill the nutritional demands of probiotics, which, as we have seen, are living bacteria. Some good examples of prebiotic foods are artichokes, leeks, onions, garlic, asparagus, bananas, legumes, honey, oats, and lentils. Prebiotics help gut health, which in turn maximizes the effectiveness of the immune system.[1]

Your food plan is a powerful weapon in the fight for optimal gut health. One of the important ways this happens is with the right balance of gut bacteria. As we have discussed previously, the Standard American Diet is not helpful in creating a favorable microbiome. The prevalence of processed carbohydrates, bad fats, and artificial ingredients in the SAD helps to create an environment where unfavorable bugs can thrive. The foods that you eat interact with the gut microbiome to create favorable or unfavorable metabolites. We can reduce the production of harmful gut metabolites through diet by replacing low-fiber foods with high-fiber ones, cutting sugar consumption, increasing diversity in food selections, and reducing overall fat intake.

When I met with Bill, I asked him to start by taking a pre- and probiotic daily. Within weeks, he developed more normal bowel movements, but he also saw improvement in his overall health. In our next meeting, we took it a step further, and along with his probiotic supplement I guided him in creating a food plan to help his overall health. He stopped buying packaged meals and learned to cook in his kitchen. Now Bill hardly ate at fast-food restaurants. He was on his way to terrific gut health.

Ultimately the results were remarkable. I have seen it time and again—the use of probiotics has been shown to help stroke recovery,[2] which is just what happened with Bill. He was quite pleased, not only with the improvement in his GI health but also with his overall well-being.

TARGETING INFLAMMATORY GUT CELLS TO SUPPORT THE MICROBIOME

Recent studies on mice provide peer-reviewed evidence for the results I saw with Bill and hold promise for using diet to reduce post-stroke inflammation. Therapies that target the gut can be used to stop the activation and migration of specific intestinal cells that cause a breach in the blood-brain barrier.

So how does this affect stroke recovery? "Big picture: seeing a persistent, chronic change 28 days after a stroke associated with this increase in some of the negative bacteria means that this could negatively affect brain function and behavior. Ultimately, this could slow or prevent post-stroke recovery," says researcher Candice Brown.[3]

Brown and Brichacek's study, which we introduced in Chapter 4, could lead to new therapeutic options for stroke patients. "If it ends up being that the gut influences the repair of the brain, maybe our stroke treatments shouldn't just be focused on what we can do for the brain. Maybe we need to think about what we can do for the gut," says Brichacek.[4]

As with my patient Bill, we have to address gut health in addition to the traditional treatments for stroke. Ischemic stroke can result in disruption of the gut barrier and movement of gut bacteria outside the gut.[5] Gut bacteria diversity also decreases after stroke. Increased amounts of bacteria in the family *Enterobacteriaceae* have been associated with poor stroke outcomes, possibly by increasing systematic inflammation and worsening brain damage.[6] These types of data give us opportunities to potentially alter outcomes after stroke by changing the microbiome of the stroke patient. We may have other therapeutic targets for improving the lives of those stricken with one of the deadliest diseases on our planet.

EATING TO PREVENT STROKE

Nutrition is an important pillar when it comes to being a health hero, and especially when it comes to preventing stroke. The foods we consume need to protect and strengthen the microbiome, in part so that we can fortify the blood-brain barrier. Because gut microbiota can influence stroke outcomes, as we saw with Bill, it is especially important to pay attention to probiotic intake. One of the most efficient ways to change the microbiome before and after stroke is to increase our intake of fermented foods, which, as we know, are powerful catalysts for the microbiome. Recent animal studies have shown that, in particular, the two most common probiotics—*Bifidobacterium breve* and *Bifidobacterium longum*—have therapeutic potential in ischemic stroke.[7] These foods are especially important as we age and our risk for stroke and disease of the brain statistically increases.[8]

Make fermented foods a regular part of your dietary routine—once or twice each day. Especially important are short-chain fatty acids, postbiotics found in fermented foods like kefir,

FERMENTED FOODS CONTAINING THE PROBIOTIC *BIFIDOBACTERIUM*

- Buttermilk
- Cheeses: Swiss, provolone, Gouda, cheddar, Edam, Gruyere
- Cottage cheese
- Kefir
- Kimchi
- Kombucha
- Miso
- Sauerkraut
- Sour pickles
- Sourdough bread
- Tempeh
- Red wine, in moderation
- Yogurt (made from milk or soy)

Carefully read food labels and look for names of specific bacteria as well as terms like "live cultures" and "contains probiotics."

tempeh, and kimchi, which help healthy bacteria flourish. Recent animal studies have indicated that "microbiota-derived SCFAs modulate poststroke recovery via effects on systemic and brain resident immune cells."[9] This is promising because it suggests that SCFAs are powerful regenerators of neuronal plasticity

WILL A BANANA A DAY KEEP STROKE AWAY?

According to the American Academy of Neurology and other recent studies, inadequate amounts of potassium in the diet are associated with a greater risk of death from stroke.[10] Bananas are a good source of potassium, providing about 420 mg (12 percent of the minimum daily requirement) per serving, but consider adding supplements or other foods high in potassium, such as:

- Acorn squash
- Avocados
- Baked potatoes with skin
- Dark leafy greens, like kale and spinach
- Dried apricots
- White beans
- Yogurt

So be sure to get enough potassium daily, especially if you are taking diuretics, which are often prescribed for hypertension (and thus for people at higher risk of stroke) and which can deplete your body's potassium.

at a structural level after stroke—in other words, consuming postbiotics may help restore the brain after stroke and become an important therapy in recovery.

MAGNESIUM AND STROKE

Maintaining optimal magnesium stores is good for health in general. Research has linked magnesium deficiencies to various chronic diseases, including type 2 diabetes, heart disease, high blood pressure, and stroke—to which I would add Alzheimer's and ADHD.[11] The mineral is crucial for regulating more than 300 enzymes in the body and is involved in essential functions such as muscle control, energy production, transmission of electrical impulses, and detoxification. By raising your body's magnesium levels, you can potentially improve or prevent those health conditions, especially if you were deficient.

This is especially important when it comes to stroke. Recent research has indicated that increasing magnesium intake may be

TAKE A BATH!

When you immerse your body in a bath enriched with Epsom salts, the magnesium ions in the salt may be absorbed through the skin. Once absorbed, the magnesium ions can enter the bloodstream, increasing the body's internal magnesium stores. Patients have even reported to me that absorbing magnesium through the skin in this manner can relieve constipation.

a crucial component of both prevention and treatment, especially in high-risk individuals.[12] So be sure to eat magnesium-rich foods, especially those that simultaneously nourish the microbiome, like black beans, leafy greens, whole grains, nuts, and

IMPROVING SLEEP HYGIENE

As we know, sleep impacts inflammation, which impacts our gut and brain (and vice versa), so do your best to get a good night's sleep.

- Maintain a consistent sleep schedule to promote healthy sleep patterns, and do your best to keep as close to it as possible on weekends. Your body does not know whether it is Sunday or Wednesday.
- Avoid consuming heavy meals, caffeine, or alcohol close to bedtime. Instead, opt for a light and balanced meal earlier in the evening, and consider replacing caffeinated drinks with herbal teas or decaffeinated options.
- Remember the Five Pillars and practice relaxation techniques such as meditation or deep breathing before sleep to promote better sleep quality.
- Monitor your sleep posture and adjust as needed to ensure optimal comfort and alignment.
- Consult a healthcare professional if you experience persistent sleep issues, such as insomnia or excessive daytime sleepiness.

avocados. If needed, you can add a magnesium supplement at the direction of your healthcare team.

THE FUTURE: ZONULIN AND MORE

Each person has a unique gut microbiome, which makes it difficult to develop one-size-fits-all treatments and prescriptions for gut dysfunction. We are just now developing diagnostic techniques that can identify a person's microbiome signature. Although these are not yet perfect, such techniques could eventually be revolutionary in improving gut health and lowering the risk of stroke.

For instance, tests for zonulin, a protein found in the intestines and liver and a biomarker of increased gut permeability, show promise in measuring the extent of leaky gut syndrome.[13] Tests can measure gut function and microbiome content and offer diet and supplement suggestions to improve gut health. You can obtain these tests under your healthcare team's supervision or by using at-home tests (brand names include Ombre and Viome). We are now able to diagnose specific microbiome patterns in our patients and understand their strengths and weaknesses. Not everyone requires the same supplement or food; while I might not need more broccoli, for example, you might. We are able to identify the types of bacteria that are deficient or present in abundance, giving us clues about risk for certain diseases.

Just like a calcium score may predict cardiac disease risk or a suspicious mammogram can alert you to a breast tumor, the microbial signature could be a warning sign for a future event.

As clinicians, we may be able to avert a health catastrophe by analyzing a stool sample.

These and other emerging treatments based on the relationship between gut health and stroke may change how we both prevent strokes and manage post-stroke recovery. The future is indeed bright, with the possibility of decreasing the burden of disease caused by this killer we call stroke.

MIND-BODY PRACTICES AND DECREASING CORTISOL

As we saw in Chapter 2, stress and gut health are connected. More stress means more cortisol in our bloodstreams, and more stress leads to increased inflammation, dysregulated blood pressure, spikes in blood sugar, and difficulty resting or bouncing back after physical or emotional challenges. In a vicious circle, excessive amounts of stress hormones and the resulting inflammation can reshape the microbiome, encouraging the "bad" bacteria that exacerbate our response to stress.

A key to decreasing cortisol levels, important in preventing stroke or during recovery, is one of the Five Pillars—spirituality. Myriad studies spanning many religions affirm again and again that spiritual practice, be it prayer, yogic heartfulness meditation, other forms of meditation and prayer, and mindfulness-based stress reduction (MBSR), decreases the body's production of stress hormones, including cortisol.[14] And I've seen in my practice how lowering our cortisol levels—especially in conjunction with other preventative actions like diet and exercise—means a lower risk of stroke.

After a stroke, patients often suffer from post-stroke depression (PSD). There is increasing evidence leading to a correlation between the presence of certain gut microbiota and the development of brain diseases like stroke, Parkinson's, and Alzheimer's via the gut-brain axis. Comparing the microbiomes of healthy and stroke-affected rats shows that the gut microbiome may also be a factor in the development of PSD.[15]

TRY MINDFULNESS-BASED STRESS REDUCTION PRACTICE

Scientists continue to gather data on the mind's impact on the microbiome, especially when it comes to cortisol levels and mindfulness-based stress reduction.[16] There are several basic MBSR techniques, including body scans (in which "neutral attention" is progressively directed toward sensations throughout our bodies) and concentrated attention on breathing while meditating or during our everyday activities.[17] What they have in common is acceptance and a nonreactive attitude toward the experiences of each moment.

Use this simple five-minute meditation practice to experiment on yourself and see if you experience a decrease in your stress levels:

- Sit in a comfortable position in a chair or on the floor. Keep your back straight, your hands resting easily in your lap.

THE FIVE PILLARS AND CHANGING THE COURSE OF STROKE

Especially with stroke and its devastating consequences, the instinct may be to react with, "Oh my gosh, there's nothing I can do. It's time to give up." Remember, though, that having a purpose can genuinely change the outcome of a stroke—I

- Allow your body to relax and pay attention to the sensations as it does so. Focus on any spots of agitation or tightness as you breathe into and release them.
- Follow your natural—not forced—breath. Inhale, exhale, inhale . . . As you focus on your breathing, you will probably notice thoughts arising or your mind wandering. As you do, label them as "thoughts" or "wandering" and gently return your attention to your breathing.
- Silently continue with this practice—breathing, noticing the mind, and returning to the simplicity of the breath—for about five minutes. You might enjoy it so much that five minutes will easily become ten.

have seen it make a difference. Once you have returned to your purpose, which might be as simple as eating with a spoon or as radical as being able to drive a car, everything else follows. Doctors will often tell you that brain function cannot be restored or preserved even after the first year, but it really can be possible for several years. My dad was living proof of this. If we had given up after six months or a year, we would not have seen the progress that he made in years two and three and the quality of life that resulted.

FOODS THAT HAVE BEEN SHOWN TO HELP PREVENT AND REDUCE THE EFFECT OF STROKE

- Beans and other legumes
- Beets and other purplish foods
- Fermented foods
- Foods rich in potassium and magnesium, such as spinach and bananas
- Ginger
- Melon
- Oatmeal
- Prunes
- Soybeans
- Sweet and white potatoes (with their skins)
- Tomatoes

Our family became health heroes, rallying around my beloved father after his stroke. My sister, my mom, and I, along with my wife, did all we could to help him thrive. Someone was always present in the hospital, the rehabilitation center, and at home. We understood the critical importance of community and tribe in his recovery.

My sister and I spent many afternoons attempting to help my father exercise and become as ambulatory as possible, as we realized that movement was fundamental in having Dad reach his potential. We were a fixture in the rehabilitation center, working with the therapists to help him take one more step.

We also did everything possible to ensure that he got the best possible nutrition. After his stroke, my dad was quite a picky eater, and he developed a fondness for the nutritional puddings you can buy in grocery stores. Although filled with calories and

THE MOST IMPORTANT THINGS TO DO FOR YOUR GUT TO PREVENT STROKE

- Decrease inflammation by changing the microbiome, using pre- and probiotics.
- Eat a gut-healthy diet rich in potassium, magnesium, and foods that sustain the microbiome.
- Remember the Five Pillars. Nutrition, movement, purpose, community, and spirituality can not only give us peace of mind but also help change our gut.

protein, these puddings contain significant amounts of processed carbohydrates and probably were not the best choice. If we had the knowledge sixteen years ago that we have now, perhaps we could have tested his stool to determine his microbiome signature. That might have helped us attack any adverse bacteria with the right food and even the right probiotics. And maybe, as a result, my dad could have had a better outcome.

In writing this book, I want to empower those who are in the position that my family was in. I want to offer tools for families to help their loved ones prevent strokes and disability, and limit these disabilities after a stroke.

CHAPTER SIX

HOW GUT HEALTH CONTRIBUTES TO ALZHEIMER'S DISEASE

I have known Mark, an exemplary high school principal in a school of 1,200 students, for sixteen years. An astute, gregarious man and a sharp dresser, he always dons a sophisticatedly coordinated outfit appropriate for the season. He is a sharp man, inside and out.

Over the years, Mark has visited me in my office for help treating irritable bowel syndrome and gastroesophageal reflux disease, commonly known as GERD. As put together as Mark is on the outside, he occasionally suffers from stress when dealing with staffing issues, troubled parents, and challenging students. When he is under duress, his symptoms worsen, and that is when he comes to see me.

One summer day, Mark was seated in my office. Distant, pensive, and almost sad, he was not himself. When I asked what was on his mind, he told me he had been given the diagnosis of Alzheimer's, and he was terrified. This smart, witty, respected leader was now having difficulty with simple tasks, ones he had been able to complete effortlessly just a few years earlier.

At sixty-eight, Mark had not previously battled any serious health crises and was active, enjoying the outdoors in northern Michigan with his wife. But Alzheimer's was changing this. His friends had begun to notice Mark's cognitive decline, making their social engagements trying, almost uncomfortable. His gut issues, which manifested as uncontrolled diarrhea, bloating, and belching, had overtaken his life, limiting him significantly.

Most folks would call Mark healthy. He ate a fairly nutritious diet, apart from the occasional french fries and ice cream, and maintained a good weight. From his outward appearance, he looked well. However, his brain health was failing.

Mark is a prime example of how someone who has been sharp as a tack, looks healthy, and has no serious medical issues can fall prey to a devastating neurodegenerative disorder. And he is not alone. In my experience, many others who develop Alzheimer's share his profile.

Historically, medical professionals have identified several risk factors for Alzheimer's. Genetics is one. But other conditions seemingly unrelated to brain health, several of which—in some cases—are more influenced by lifestyle choices than DNA, have also been connected to the onset of Alzheimer's. These include diabetes, obesity, and heart disease. Each of these conditions can develop via a common mechanism within the body, one that involves inflammation. Now, researchers are beginning to see another consistent pattern: It turns out that people with Alzheimer's also have an unhealthy microbiome. Even folks genetically predisposed to Alzheimer's disease seem to have an unbalanced microbiome. Gut dysbiosis is turning out to be a common denominator among all these conditions.[1]

We will look more closely at the risk factors for Alzheimer's and see how each of these might contribute to leaky gut, inflammation, and neurodegeneration. But first, what is Alzheimer's, and why are so many people afraid that they might be a candidate?

WHAT IS ALZHEIMER'S DISEASE?

Alzheimer's disease is one of the most feared medical conditions—and for good reason. Over time, it creates chaos in the brain, causing neurons to misfire or die off and the thoughts and memories once associated with them to vanish. As neurons die,

SYMPTOMS OF ALZHEIMER'S

Symptoms of Alzheimer's may include difficulty with:

- Simple, familiar tasks.
- Memory (especially recalling recent information) and problem-solving.
- Time/place recognition.
- Comprehension of images and spatial relationships.
- Communication.
- Retracing steps: *How did I get here?*
- Family, work, and social activities.
- Personality changes, some the direct consequence of Alzheimer's, plus depression, anxiety, and anger at having dementia.

cognitive abilities decline, dementia sets in, and the brain itself begins to shrink.

Alzheimer's changes everything—how we get through the day, whether we are able to work, our social life, all our relationships. And it diminishes and ultimately destroys skill sets we once took for granted—the ability to tend a beautiful garden, play the piano, drive a car, pay the bills, make dinner, or even use a lawn mower.

This disease is devastating to individuals, most of whom are aware, at least initially, that they are losing their faculties. It is trying and heartbreaking for family members to watch and endure, especially since most Alzheimer's patients are cared for at home by a loved one.[2] Aggressive and sometimes violent outbursts are not unusual. A tendency to wander, coupled with an inability to remember how they got someplace, can make those with AD extremely difficult to care for. Silver Alerts, sent out by a public notification system that exists in most states primarily to help find missing Alzheimer's family members, are on the rise, with thousands being issued each year.

What is often most heartbreaking is that patients are no longer recognizable to their loved ones. Their physical features may not change, but the personality and behaviors of patients with Alzheimer's are forever altered, breaking their spirit and the spirits of those who love them. This is the price and burden of Alzheimer's.

There are several different types of dementia, each category sharing a common denominator. Alzheimer's is the most common, affecting more than 50 million adults worldwide. In the United States, Alzheimer's is the seventh-leading cause of death.[3] While Western countries have an increased incidence of Alzheimer's compared to the rest of the world, the percentage of people afflicted is accelerating and expanding into more populations where it was once uncommon. Despite intense efforts by the medical community to find a solution, the problem is growing, as more people—usually between the ages of sixty-five and eighty—are diagnosed with Alzheimer's.

Alzheimer's is characterized by a buildup in the brain of beta-amyloid, a protein that, if allowed to proliferate unchecked, forms into toxic, sticky plaques that interfere with neuronal pathways. Another protein called tau, which is shaped more like a loose piece of string, naturally exists within neurons, binding with structures called microtubules. But in Alzheimer's, tau separates from its host and binds instead with other tau. If enough instances of this occur, the threads of tau knot up with one another, much like the chain on a necklace that has been recklessly tossed into a purse or jewelry box, and form what are known as neurofibrillary tangles within a neuron.[4]

These plaques and tangles are highly disruptive. Like a hodgepodge of cars and buses and delivery trucks in a downtown traffic jam, the combination of beta-amyloid plaques and neurofibrillary tangles prevents much of anything from getting through. Most notably, they block the communication signals between neurons so essential to normal brain functioning. Importantly, they also trigger an immune response.

The immune system is, as we know, designed to protect the body. But in the case of Alzheimer's, something goes awry. Normally, immune cells called microglia, the brain's housekeepers, act as scavengers within the central nervous system, cleaning up toxins and debris such as dead cells that might interfere with brain function. They are also capable of triggering a strong inflammatory response when necessary to protect the brain from suffering damage by an invader.

In the case of Alzheimer's, researchers suggest that amyloid protein associated with the plaques activates the microglia.[5] Their first response may be effective, but as plaques and tangles are produced, the microglia get overwhelmed and begin acting erratically. At this point, the cells initially released to protect the brain are not doing so, but continue to produce inflammation.

Chronic inflammation is the crux of this brain disorder. Over the past decade, researchers have found a sustained immune response in the brain in Alzheimer's patients in reaction to the buildup of amyloid beta plaques and neurofibrillary tangles. Ultimately, the plaques, tangles, and inflammation interfere with neuronal function to the point where neurons begin to die.[6]

This damage is thought to begin years, even decades, before symptoms of Alzheimer's surface. Alzheimer's is known to first target the entorhinal cortex and hippocampus, areas of the brain associated with learning and memory. As Alzheimer's progresses, it leaves behind a path of neuronal destruction through the cerebral cortex, the part of the brain that gives us the ability to use language, to reason, and to be socially engaged. The disease eventually reaches the neocortex. In humans' evolutionary timeline, the neocortex is the newest addition to the brain and is credited with advanced functions, including sensory perception, motor commands, spatial reasoning, cognition, and language.

When inflammation reaches the neocortex, it leads to neuro-degeneration that is especially apparent in a person's behaviors. Upset, anger, and worry, for instance, are often quite common.

On average, Alzheimer's takes ten years to run its course. And science has not yet found an effective treatment, much less learned how to reverse the neuropathology of Alzheimer's—to undo the tangled tau or completely dissolve the sticky amyloid plaques. Once someone is diagnosed with Alzheimer's, there is no turning back the clock.

Alzheimer's has no known cure partly because we cannot say with 100 percent certainty what causes it. Several cognition-enhancing medications are available (Donepezil, also known as Aricept, rivastigmine, or Exelon, and galantamine, or Reminyl) to improve thinking and memory, but they seem to have mostly temporary effects. Aducanumab, which was approved in 2021 via the FDA's Accelerated Approval Program, was a "disease-modifying" drug available to treat Alzheimer's. Aducanumab was used to treat mild and moderate cases but was removed from the market in January 2024.[7] Lecanemab is an intravenous medication used to treat mild Alzheimer's disease, and it reduces the number of amyloid-beta proteins.

Slowing progression of symptoms and attacking plaques are helpful steps, but they are not satisfying long-term solutions, because they treat the consequence of the disease rather than the root cause. Despite the nearly $3.7 billion devoted annually to Alzheimer's research in the United States alone, a treatment that would stop or reverse the progression of the disease does not yet exist.[8] This is not surprising, as the problem and the human body are both complex, and the brains of people with Alzheimer's cannot be fully investigated until after death.

Let's look at what we do know about the causes of Alzheimer's.

HOW DOES ALZHEIMER'S START?

Genetics, diabetes, obesity, and heart disease have long been associated with Alzheimer's. If a person has any of these conditions or is genetically predisposed to Alzheimer's, they are more likely to suffer from the disease. When we look at the relationship between these factors and the microbiome, we get an interesting picture: each of these can be linked to poor gut health and even specific microbe imbalances. This recent revelation is taking the scientific community down entirely new paths when it comes to Alzheimer's—treatments focused on altering the gut microbiome.

THE "ALZHEIMER'S GENE"

It is safe to say that almost anyone who has a parent who has suffered from Alzheimer's has at least one thing in common: the fear that they might carry the "Alzheimer's gene" as well.

Alzheimer's does have a genetic component, but having genes associated with the disease is not a death sentence. The genes associated with Alzheimer's are variants—genes that have permanently changed in structure. A genetic variant can be inherited when, somewhere along your ancestral lineage, a gene permanently changed and was passed on to offspring because it was present in sperm or egg cells. A genetic variant can also occur during a lifetime and not be passed on to offspring. For instance, our DNA occasionally makes a mistake when copying itself. This is more common in individuals who smoke cigarettes or are exposed to excessive (skin-cancer-causing) levels of sunlight.[9]

Genetic variants can cause disease—or not. These variants are sometimes called mutations. Even if they are able to cause disease, there is no guarantee that individuals carrying this variant *express* the associated disease. As we are learning through the study of epigenetics, whether we express some genes can be highly dependent on our environment and lifestyle. Stress and trauma, exercise, diet, and chemicals in the environment can all play a role, with the power to switch a gene on or off.

The genes associated with Alzheimer's are different for early-onset and late-onset Alzheimer's. As the names imply, the distinction between the two is the age at which a person starts noticing symptoms. Early-onset Alzheimer's occurs before age 65 and symptoms can (but rarely) occur in the third decade of life. Early onset is rare, making up only 10 percent of Alzheimer's cases, but it can be inherited in up to 15 percent of cases. If one parent develops early-onset disease, a child has a 50 percent chance of having the disease.[10]

The three known early-onset variants are *APP,* the gene that controls production of amyloid precursor protein; *PSEN1,* which encodes for the production of the protein presenilin 1; and *PSEN2,* which encodes for the protein presenilin 2. If a person expresses any of these three inherited genes, the variant will at some point begin to break down the amyloid precursor protein itself, causing the development of the beta-amyloid plaques that are so devastating to the brain.

Late-onset Alzheimer's is what most of us are familiar with, and it can begin around the time most people retire or later. It is associated with a different variant, *APOE*, which encodes for the protein called apolipoprotein E (apoE), a protein that, among other duties, helps to carry fats, also called lipids, through the bloodstream. *APOE* comes in three different forms called "alleles." We inherit two *APOE* alleles from each parent. There are three main different alleles that we can inherit, referred to as ε2, ε3, and ε4. It is here where our genetics can seem like the luck of the draw.

WHO IS AT RISK FOR ALZHEIMER'S DISEASE?

- *Age.* Most people with Alzheimer's are sixty-five and older. After age sixty-five the risk doubles every five years, and after age eighty-five, the risk reaches nearly one in three.[11]
- *Family.* Those who have a parent or sibling with Alzheimer's are more likely to develop the disease as a result of either genetics or environmental factors. This risk increases along with the number of family members who have the illness.
- *Head injury.* Links have been made between traumatic brain injury and Alzheimer's disease.[12]
- *Cardiovascular disease.* An increase in Alzheimer's risk is associated with several conditions that impair the heart and blood vessels, in particular,

APOE ε2, for instance, is thought to be protective, and so having one or more of these alleles indicates we might maintain reasonable cognitive health even well into our nineties. A University of California, Irvine, study looked at the autopsied brains and medical records of eighty-five people over age ninety who had been diagnosed with either "all-cause" dementia or Alzheimer's. The participants were selected from the 90+ Study, an initiative begun in 2003 that looks at factors contributing to the longevity of the "oldest old" by visiting and testing participants every six months. The researchers found that the brains of *APOE ε2*

heart disease, diabetes, stroke, and elevated blood pressure or cholesterol.[14]

- *Heritage.* In the United States, Latinos are about one-and-a-half times as likely as white people to develop Alzheimer's and other dementias, while African Americans are about twice as likely to have the disease.[15]
- *Acute COVID-19.* Reports of post-acute sequelae of COVID-19 (PASC, or "long" or post-acute COVID) and evidence of systemic inflammation as a driver of cognitive decline and neurodegeneration suggest that survivors of COVID-19 may be at a higher risk of developing Alzheimer's.[16]
- *Dysbiosis and leaky gut.* There appears to be a link between both early- and late-onset Alzheimer's and gut microbiome composition.[17]

carriers could show the hallmark signs of Alzheimer's—plaques and tangles—yet their cognition remained mostly intact.[13]

How *APOE ε2* protects cognition even when the brain shows signs of Alzheimer's is not entirely clear, but researchers have found that *APOE ε2* is associated with reduced amyloid-beta plaques along the neuronal pathways that are associated with Alzheimer's.[18]

Although the *ε2* allele cannot guarantee we will not get Alzheimer's, it does mean that if we do get the disease, we will likely experience it late in life and have fewer symptoms, plaques, and tangles than people who do not carry *ε2*.[19]

APOE ε4 is the allele most associated with late-onset Alzheimer's, but even if we carry the allele, it does not mean we will get Alzheimer's. As I said earlier, having a variant does not mean we will express it. About 25 percent of the population has one copy of *APOE ε4*, and only 2–3 percent carry two copies. How *ε4* contributes to the disease is not fully understood, but the more we look at the microbiome, the clearer it becomes that gut health and brain health influence each other.

APOE ε3 is the most common allele, and it seems to neither increase nor decrease the risk of getting late-onset Alzheimer's.

ALZHEIMER'S GENES AND THE GUT

Trying to make sense of the relationship among genetics, gut health, and brain health poses a bit of a chicken-or-egg conundrum. Which comes first? Do genes influence brain health and/or gut health? Or does gut health influence genetic expression and brain health? The verdict is still out, with emerging research revealing different facets of Alzheimer's pathology. Evidence suggests that the relation between Alzheimer's and gut microbiome composition is of considerable interest, and could connect poor gut health with this disease.[20]

With late-onset disease, in a study that compared the *APOE* genotypes and microbiomes of humans and genetically altered mice, researchers learned that although the microbiota of all groups was diverse, the abundance of certain microbes varied between each *APOE* genotype in humans and mice. Each *APOE* genotype, in other words, was associated with a particular gut microbiome profile. The microbiome of those with *APOE ε4* had significantly fewer butyrate-producing bacteria and short-chain fatty acids—the cells that help to maintain the integrity of the gastrointestinal barrier and protect against leaky gut.[21]

APOE is not only an indicator of how likely we are to experience Alzheimer's. *APOE* alleles are involved in several biological processes. In addition to coding for the protein apoE, which transports lipids (as mentioned earlier), *APOE* alleles are key players in what is known as lipoprotein metabolism, which involves, among other things, converting or storing fats for energy. In another study, *APOE ε4* was associated with disruptions in lipid metabolism in the brain, resulting in brain cells' inability to process fats. The resulting buildup in lipids in the brain had an adverse effect on cells, causing them to malfunction.[22] Lipids are also in direct communication with the gut microbiome through the gut-brain axis.[23] It is believed that the loss of butyrate-producing bacteria and SCFAs in *APOE ε4* carriers drives the disruption in lipid metabolism.

In a recent breakthrough animal study, researchers at Oregon Health and Science University tested whether gut health could influence whether we expressed an Alzheimer's gene. Using both wild mice and genetically engineered mice that carried the human amyloid precursor protein—the protein that when broken down creates beta-amyloid plaques—researchers looked at the behaviors and cognition of mice after six months. By observing activities such as nest building and maze running, the researchers found that the genetically engineered mice did not perform as well as their wild counterparts and linked gut microbes with the expression of some of the genetic variants associated with Alzheimer's.

By looking at the mice's fecal pellets, the researchers found that the microbiome was altered in the mice carrying the human amyloid precursor protein. Specifically, that protein altered the *Lachnospiraceae* and *Ruminococcaceae* families of microbes, both of which are beneficial bacteria and producers of butyrate.[24]

The study shows the connection between the microbiome and altered brain health—a remarkable observation, giving us the foundation for a new method of affecting this devastating illness. The researchers are following up with a study that looks at whether Alzheimer's-like symptoms can be reduced in genetically altered mice by improving their diet.[25]

DIABETES, INSULIN RESISTANCE, AND OBESITY

At its core, diabetes is a metabolic problem. The food we eat enters the intestines, where it is broken down into its basic components—protein, fats, and carbohydrates (sugars such as glucose) to use for energy—and intentionally released via the gastrointestinal barrier into the bloodstream. The body has a hormone in place to make sure glucose makes its way from the blood into our cells: insulin, which is released by the pancreas whenever it senses the blood contains enough sugar to process. In people with diabetes, the amount of insulin available is off-kilter—either production is too low or the body has trouble using what is available. The result is excess sugar in the bloodstream while the body's cells are starved of energy. It is as if our cells were hungry sharks swimming in a sea full of fish that they cannot catch.

This lack of "cell food" is problematic. Without energy, cells will die, so they turn to the next-best source of food, fat. To make fat consumable, the liver is charged with breaking down fat into acids called ketones and then releasing them into the bloodstream. The cells now have food. But if the production of ketones is too rapid, diabetics can experience ketoacidosis, a condition in which the blood becomes too acidic. Excessive acids in the bloodstream have life-threatening consequences.

A lack of the preferred energy source (glucose) is not the only problem. Without the aid of insulin, excess sugar in the bloodstream has nowhere to go. Normally, after we eat a meal, insulin takes a few hours to move glucose into the cells and lower blood sugar levels. With diabetes, blood sugar levels stay high for extended periods and can lead to damage to the vessels that carry blood to the body's organs.

Damage to blood vessels can cause serious health consequences, including heart disease, stroke, vision loss, and kidney disease. Insulin injection can increase insulin levels and help regulate blood sugar. Insulin, oral medicines, a controlled diet, and regular exercise make up the current treatment model for this serious disease.

Like Alzheimer's, diabetes can be inherited. Type 1 diabetes usually begins in childhood or young adulthood. This version of diabetes is considered an autoimmune disease because the body's immune system attacks its own cells—in this case the cells that produce insulin. Dozens of genes are associated with type 1 diabetes, but again, having any of these genes does not mean you will necessarily express them. Lifestyle and environment matter too.

Type 2 diabetes is often connected to lifestyle and particularly diet. Being overweight or inactive can trigger insulin resistance, which is when the body does not use insulin effectively. There is also a genetic component to type 2 diabetes, especially if a person is overweight or obesity is genetic in nature. But obesity, we are learning, is not necessarily a matter of how many calories we consume versus how many we expend. And diabetes, which in most cases involves lifestyle to a large degree, may not start with problems in the pancreas. Rather, these conditions might just originate in the gut.

DIABETES, INSULIN RESISTANCE, OBESITY . . . AND GUT HEALTH

Research linking the microbiome and the development of diabetes is growing and gaining consensus. In a 2019 study, researchers showed that the production and release of certain gut metabolites—including lipopolysaccharides, short-chain fatty acids, and trimethylamine N-oxide—into the bloodstream due to gut dysbiosis and leaky gut contribute to the development of diabetes.[26]

As you may recall from Chapter 1, when LPS is released into the bloodstream, the immune system is activated, and the result is inflammation, so crucial to immune defense. We also learned that SCFAs such as butyrate, propionate, and acetate are normally protective. They result when microbes ferment fiber, and they feed the lining of the gut, keeping it durable and helping to prevent leaky gut. Gut dysbiosis, however, leads to an abnormal production of SCFAs, which impairs the gut lining and activates the inflammatory response.

TMAO is a product of the gut microbiome. Gut bacteria produce trimethylamine when digesting animal products—meat, dairy, and egg yolk. TMAO enters the bloodstream through the liver and can set off a chain reaction of physiological events that can lead to atherosclerosis, or plaques in the arteries. But it does more. In a 2019 study, TMAO was shown to disrupt glucose metabolism, an event that can lead to insulin resistance.[27]

Two years after that groundbreaking study, US and Austrian researchers made the connection between obesity and specific microbes important to how we metabolize glucose and lipids. To look into the effects of diet on the microbiome and, subsequently, the development of type 2 diabetes, the scientists fed one group of mice a regular mouse diet. They fed the other group food consistent with a Western diet. Not surprisingly, mice on the Western diet developed glucose intolerance and insulin resistance. They were on a fast track to developing type 2 diabetes.

After studying the fecal pellets for insight into the microbiome of each group of mice, the researchers singled out four bacteria that either helped or harmed the mice: *Lactobacillus gasseri* was beneficial, while *Romboutsia ilealis* and *Ruminococcus gnavus* were harmful. Interestingly, when they compared the microbiomes and body mass indexes (BMIs) of humans, people who had significant numbers of the "good" bacteria were a healthier weight than those who had significant numbers of the "bad" bacteria. The conclusion? Those mice with the "bad" bacteria were less protected from the harmful effects of a Western diet. In fact, about 80 percent of those who had higher levels of *Romboutsia ilealis* were obese.[28]

While this study was conducted on mice and not humans, the findings nonetheless could have major implications for addressing diabetes with targeted microbial treatments rather than simply asking someone to take a general probiotic. It is an exciting possibility for treating and potentially preventing such a disabling disease.

In another 2021 study, researchers found that a diverse microbiome rich in bacteria known to produce butyrate helped protect people against developing insulin resistance and type 2 diabetes. This study was significant in that it looked at stool samples of more than 2,000 people—possibly the largest study to date to look specifically at gut health and diabetes.[29]

HEART DISEASE: WHAT YOUR DOCTOR MAY NOT TELL YOU

Most of us likely know someone who has suffered a heart attack, perhaps even in our own family. Heart disease, which includes heart attack, is the number-one killer worldwide. In the United States, it takes nearly 700,000 lives per year.[30] Coronary artery disease (CAD) is one form of heart disease, and it is the most common. CAD can include symptoms of chest pain, shortness of breath, and lightheadedness. Often the first symptom of CAD is a heart attack.

Like Alzheimer's, CAD involves plaque, only this plaque accumulates on the inside walls of arteries that supply blood to the heart. Its source is not the amyloid precursor protein but rather deposits of cholesterol and other substances. As the deposits build, the pathway within the artery narrows, leaving less room for blood to flow freely. This narrowing and "hardening" of the arteries due to plaque is known as atherosclerosis.

Because it slows blood flow to the heart, atherosclerosis is troublesome. If severe enough, plaque buildup can block an artery entirely. But there is another problem that you may not hear about: inflammation within the arteries.

Inflammation within the arteries has been linked to the gut, specifically to a group of cells known as mononuclear phagocytes (MNPs).[31] While these cells are found throughout the body, they play a prominent role within the intestine when it comes to maintaining homeostasis within the gut and regulating immune responses and therefore inflammation. Increased inflammation in the gut can result in increased inflammation throughout the body, including the arteries.

Most people do not think of inflammation as contributing to a blocked artery, but inflammation greatly increases your risk of heart attack by damaging the walls of arteries. Inflammation can also lead to a heart attack by increasing the rate of plaque growth and loosening plaques that can then trigger blood clots in your arteries.

High blood pressure and smoking are known risk factors for heart disease. At the risk of sounding like a broken record, diabetes, obesity, a Western diet (SAD), and lack of physical activity are other contributors.

HEART DISEASE AND GUT HEALTH

Researchers are now going so far as to say that we may have the cause of atherosclerosis backward. Instead of cholesterol being the first to arrive on the scene—collecting in and hardening the arteries with plaque—inflammation in the blood vessels precedes the cholesterol.[32] When "bad" bacteria in the gut produce chemicals such as TMAO, LPS, and excessive amounts of SCFAs, damage the gastrointestinal barrier, and escape into the bloodstream, where the chemicals will eventually land is anyone's guess. But wherever they land, the inflammatory immune response is sure to follow.

Because these "inflammation magnets" are transported by blood vessels, our veins and arteries often bear the brunt of the inflammation. Inflammation in blood vessels, we now know, damages the vessel walls, decreasing their ability to function. This in turn affects the vessel's elasticity. This inflammation can also increase the risk of plaque to grow and break off, triggering a heart attack. High levels of TMAO, in particular, have been associated with a cardiovascular event.

MICROBIOME RESEARCH AND ALZHEIMER'S

The lines between disease states, such as heart disease and diabetes, and the role they play in whether we will develop Alzheimer's are often blurred, with some debate surrounding what factors lead to the chemical reactions in the brain that lead to the hallmark symptoms of beta-amyloid plaque and neurofibrillary tangles. But one thing is becoming increasingly clear: each of the other health conditions associated with Alzheimer's can also be associated with poor gut health.

The overlap in disease states and pathologies leading to Alzheimer's is significant enough to merit our close attention. While we do not know everything that contributes to someone developing Alzheimer's, we do know that inflammation is significant. The more we learn about the microbiome, the more we can associate the inflammation so pronounced in Alzheimer's and other dementias with the inflammation created by poor gut health. TMAO, for instance, has been found in cerebrospinal fluid—the clear fluid that cushions the spine and brain. Where there is TMAO, there is inflammation.

With this knowledge, we are poised to make changes that can affect the course of Alzheimer's. With subtle but significant changes made every day, we can fight a killer. Using the gut as our tool, we can help optimize our brain and better manage and even prevent Alzheimer's. But how?

CHAPTER SEVEN

CHANGING THE COURSE OF ALZHEIMER'S DISEASE

Once he was diagnosed with Alzheimer's disease, my patient Mark visited me several times during that summer and fall. I asked him to change some of his activities, including the treats he enjoyed so much. He was a great patient and "all in" on becoming a health hero, so he did not grumble too much when I said he had to avoid ice cream and french fries. His wife told me he had given the contents of his candy jar to the neighborhood kids and thrown away the jar.

Mark paid attention to the Five Pillars. Purposeful, community-based meals became part of his regimen, and he ate dinner with his family whenever he could. In consultation with his neurologist and family doctor, and in line with the recommendations I share in this chapter, Mark made changes that shaped his prescription plan. He gradually had more control of his GERD and irritable bowel syndrome symptoms and, to his family's surprise and delight, had some significant improvement in his cognitive skills, regaining the ability to perform some of the tasks he had not been able to handle just a few months earlier. Mark and his family were happy and hopeful about his future.

Gut care is a novel approach to Alzheimer's care, but it is a method that could drastically alter our treatment and prevention of the disease. Many who suffer from this devastating illness seldom receive hope for a brighter future. By targeting gut health, these patients and their families may have another means to address Alzheimer's with simple, effective principles that can impact this neurodegenerative disease and their whole health as well.

THE ALZHEIMER'S GUT

Evidence that the gut microbiome and Alzheimer's are connected is mounting. Researchers in Ireland, England, and Italy have recently reported that "Alzheimer's symptoms can be transferred to a healthy young organism via the gut microbiota, confirming a causal role of gut microbiota in Alzheimer's disease."[1] This data is quite valuable, because it confirms what we have suspected for a long time—the bidirectional communication between the gut and the brain when it comes to Alzheimer's disease.

Leading up to this report, in a 2022 study, researchers from King's College in London analyzed the blood and stool samples of sixty-eight people with Alzheimer's disease (AD) and sixty-eight people who showed no signs of dementia. The "Alzheimer's gut" was distinct, with an increase in the number of inflammation markers.[2] This follows up on findings that the gut microbiomes of people with preclinical AD (indicated by altered brain amyloid and tau proteins) had a different composition from those of healthy individuals.[3]

Other recent research has shown that rats implanted with stools from people with Alzheimer's did not grow as many nerve cells as rats in the control group. And early trials are beginning to suggest that treating brain stem cells with blood from Alzheimer's patients can disrupt nerve cell growth, leading researchers to conclude that inflammation in the bloodstream associated with gut metabolites can affect the brain.[4]

All of this is to say that when it comes to Alzheimer's disease, the research on the gut-brain axis is evolving rapidly, but in my opinion there is one thing about which there is no doubt: there is a definite connection.

FROM INDIA TO ITALY: REVERSING INFLAMMATION WITH NUTRITION

This connection is something I have suspected for quite some time. In my practice I have seen many patients with Alzheimer's who have eaten the standard Western diet for their entire lives and, like Mark, have fallen victim to this disease. If we look around the globe at other cultures with different diets and compare incidences of Alzheimer's, we begin to see a correlation.

Take India, for instance. Until recently, when the Western diet became more prevalent, India was cited as having one of the lowest rates of Alzheimer's in the world.[5] In northern India, fewer than 1 percent of those over the age of fifty-five had Alzheimer's—far below the worldwide and US averages.[6] Though India does not excel in high blood pressure control or diabetes control, most Indians regularly cook with turmeric, a well-known anti-inflammatory agent.

As discussed earlier, turmeric is a potent anti-inflammatory agent. A great tool for achieving gut health, it has been used for centuries in Asia and is now popular worldwide. The active ingredient in turmeric is gut-friendly curcumin, which has been shown to improve intestinal barrier function and combat intestinal permeability (leaky gut). Turmeric also works with the gut microbiome to decrease inflammation, which is what makes it well suited to help in the fight against diseases such as Alzheimer's.[7]

When I recommended turmeric to Mark, at first he was apprehensive, but eventually he discovered it was quite easy to incorporate turmeric into his diet. Turmeric does not significantly change the taste of the food and is caffeine free, low in calories, and rich in nutrients. It can be mixed into your favorite drinks, including tea, cocoa, and smoothies. I add it to scrambled eggs, lentils, and veggies. Turmeric is absorbed well when taken with food, especially foods containing fat and with a dash of black pepper.

Although turmeric is a fantastic addition, changing one thing about a diet is not enough, so it is important to consider a lifelong way of eating that can help reduce inflammation and decrease brain atrophy.

THE MEDITERRANEAN DIET

When it comes to Alzheimer's disease and helping the microbiome thrive, I tend to recommend the Mediterranean diet to my patients because it has been shown to be effective in decreasing inflammation, which is so important in general and especially when it comes to neurodegenerative disease.[8]

This accessible diet, which is easy for patients to adopt, is based on traditional foods consumed by European cultures around the Mediterranean—particularly in Greece and Italy—and is marked by being low in saturated fat and higher in vegetable oils. Although exact definitions vary, they all include guidelines for consumption of extra-virgin (cold-pressed) olive oil, vegetables including leafy greens, fruits, whole grains, nuts, and beans/legumes. There is moderate to low consumption of fish and other meat, cheese, yogurt, and red wine, and low intakes of eggs and sweets.[9] To this I add herbs and spices and recommend that red meat be eaten only rarely if at all. I emphasize that patients (whether they have Alzheimer's or not) should avoid eating processed meat or any highly processed food, refined grains and oils, foods with added sugars, and beverages sweetened with sugar.

As they make the transition to my interpretation of the Mediterranean diet, I encourage patients to begin by making it a point to eat:

- Beans
- Fiber-rich foods or a supplement like psyllium husks
- Fruits
- Legumes
- Nuts and seeds
- Oily fish, in moderation
- Olives and olive oil

- Probiotic and prebiotic foods like yogurt and bananas
- Some spices, such as ginger and turmeric
- Vegetables, especially leafy greens

Simultaneously, I encourage them to avoid:

- Alcohol
- Foods with excessive amounts of sugar or salt
- Hydrogenated palm or coconut oils
- Pre-made desserts
- Processed foods

Along with this, depending on the patient's palate, I recommend they add in other anti-inflammatory foods, especially:

- Avocados
- Organic berries, cherries, and grapes
- Broccoli
- Fermented foods
- Green tea
- Mushrooms
- And, of course, turmeric

SUPPLEMENTS

Transforming our diet seldom happens overnight, so as patients are making the transition into an anti-inflammatory diet, over-the-counter supplements can be helpful in altering the microbiome in the gut, especially:

- Probiotics like *Lactobacillus,* which has been shown to improve cognitive function.
- The postbiotic butyrate (discussed earlier), which decreases inflammation.
- Gamma-aminobutyric acid (GABA), which can reduce anxiety and depression associated with Alzheimer's by modulating dysfunction in the gut-brain axis.
- Vitamin D.

Probiotics. Just as with stroke and Parkinson's disease, pre- and probiotics are essential to enhancing and maintaining the microbiome. Diets rich in pre- and probiotics (found naturally in fermented foods such as pickles and sauerkraut, leading to decreased intestinal permeability and inflammation) can bring immediate and dramatic improvements in gut discomfort and prevent further damage to the brain. How does this connect to Alzheimer's in particular? Due to the increased health of the gut, there is decreased inflammation and thus decreased factors that can cause inflammation throughout the body, including Alzheimer's. If eating fermented foods is not an option, I recommend both pre- and probiotic supplements.

Butyrate. Studies are finding that the effects of the compound sodium butyrate can improve the pathological status of Alzheimer's disease.[10] Butyrate does this by regulating gene expression in the brain, where it has several beneficial effects on neurodegenerative disorders. Butyrate can be produced in the gut by eating copious amounts of dietary fiber. It is also present in butter and Parmesan cheese. However, the healthiest and most efficient way to introduce sodium butyrate to the gut is by regularly eating beans and legumes. If eating a bean-rich high-fiber diet proves to be difficult, butyrate supplements are readily available.

GABA. Gamma-aminobutyric acid is a neurotransmitter in our brain that slows down or blocks specific signals in the central nervous system and is known to produce a calming effect. It can be found in some fermented foods, including miso and tempeh, as well as black and green tea, brown rice, soybeans, mushrooms, sweet potatoes, sprouted grains, and cruciferous vegetables. It hasn't been conclusively determined how effective GABA supplements are at permeating the blood-brain barrier, so as always, food is the first choice, but since early trials on mice have shown some promise and GABA may help to relieve the anxiety and confusion related to Alzheimer's as well, it is a supplement I consider giving under the appropriate circumstances.[11]

Vitamin D. Vitamin D is key to all-around health, especially gut health. Note that poor gut health can be an indicator of inflammatory bowel disease among others.[12]

We get vitamin D from fattier foods, oily fish, and egg yolks as well as fortified beverages and sun exposure, so it's a supplement I frequently recommend, especially because the variables of food and time outdoors in sunny weather can be hard to control. When it comes to Alzheimer's disease prevention and treatment, vitamin D is crucial. Not only is it widely accepted that vitamin D decreases inflammation,[13] but a deficiency has already been linked to the onset and progression of many neurological diseases, including Alzheimer's.[14]

INTERMITTENT FASTING

Although nutrition is one of the Five Pillars that health heroes rely on, sometimes it is not what we put into our gut but what we *do not* that can make all the difference. As our understanding of nutrition and the human body grows, fasting methods have evolved, leading to various approaches, each with its advantages. Among these, the intermittent fasting method stands out as particularly noteworthy because it has been shown to reduce inflammation—one of the biggest culprits in Alzheimer's disease, as we know.[15]

In a recent article on the effects of intermittent fasting on cognitive health and Alzheimer's disease, Dr. Alby Elias, senior fellow of the Academic Unit for Psychiatry of Old Age, Department of Psychiatry, University of Melbourne, wrote, "Physiological alterations associated with fasting have profound implications for pathological mechanisms associated with dementias, particularly Alzheimer's disease. Compared with ad libitum feeding (in which food is available at all times), caloric restriction in animals was associated with a reduction in β-amyloid accumulation, which is the cardinal pathological marker of Alzheimer's disease. Animal studies have demonstrated synaptic adaptations in the hippocampus and enhanced cognitive function after fasting, consistent with these theoretical frameworks. Furthermore, vascular dysfunction plays a crucial role in Alzheimer's disease pathology, and intermittent fasting promotes vascular health."

He concluded, "These observations lead to a hypothesis that intermittent fasting over the years will potentially reverse or delay the pathological process in Alzheimer's disease."[16] What a remarkable tool to add to our health hero toolkit!

When it comes to intermittent fasting, the recommended time without eating is sixteen hours. It is a simple principle: fasting—not introducing anything except unsweetened beverages into our gut for sixteen consecutive hours and then eating during an eight-hour window. This fasting pattern leverages the body's transition from using available glucose for energy to tapping into fat stores, resulting in potential weight loss and improved fat metabolism. In the sixteen-hour fasting window, the body enters a state of ketosis, where fat breakdown becomes a primary energy source. This shift is associated with various health benefits, including enhanced insulin sensitivity, which is crucial for regulating blood sugar levels.

Moreover, the sixteen-hour fasting period may stimulate autophagy, a process in which cells remove damaged components, promoting cellular renewal and having potential longevity benefits. The eight-hour eating window allows individuals to fulfill their nutritional needs and enjoy balanced meals, making it a practical approach for many.

If implemented correctly, intermittent fasting can boost metabolism, increase energy levels, and lead to potential health improvements. By increasing the diversity of the microbiome, intermittent fasting can yield benefits in gut health and decrease inflammation. Recent studies have shown that the microbiome remodeling that can occur with intermittent fasting can help diseases such as hypertension and obesity.[17] Thus, intermittent fasting may be an effective method in the fight against Alzheimer's via its effects on gut health.

However, while the benefits of intermittent fasting can be profound, it is important to remember that it may not be suitable for everyone.

- Intermittent fasting is part of a holistic approach—a lifestyle that includes balanced nutrition, regular exercise, and sufficient rest complements the gains from intermittent fasting. Mindful eating and understanding your body's signals further contribute to a successful intermittent journey.
- Selecting the right sixteen-hour fasting window requires careful consideration to ensure it aligns with your lifestyle and goals. Eating patterns should complement your daily routine and preferences while optimizing the benefits of intermittent fasting.
- Begin by evaluating your daily schedule and identifying periods when you can comfortably abstain from consuming calories for sixteen hours. Some individuals prefer to start their fasting window in the evening, while others find it more suitable to start their fast during the morning hours. Listen to your body and choose a time frame that allows for consistency and adherence, enabling you to reap the rewards of this fasting approach effectively.
- Overeating can strain the body,[18] making periodic fasting essential for allowing the body to reset and maintain proper function.

- The 16:8 diet allows you to drink calorie-free beverages like water and unsweetened tea and coffee during the sixteen-hour fasting period. Regular fluid intake is crucial to prevent dehydration. Most people who follow the 16:8 plan abstain from food at night and for part of the morning and evening. There are no restrictions on the types or amounts of food (in moderation) you can eat during the eight-hour window. This flexibility makes the plan relatively easy to follow.

- The 16:8 intermittent fasting method does not dictate specific food choices, but it is advisable to prioritize healthy foods and minimize junk food intake. Choosing organic or locally sourced ingredients helps prevent toxin buildup from harmful preservatives and pesticides, promoting better health. Even if you're doing intermittent fasting, it is crucial to avoid foods high in fats, sugars, and refined carbohydrates.

WHY FASTING SEEMS TO WORK: LYSOSOMES

Research into the causes of dementia and Alzheimer's disease has often focused on the buildup of tangles and plaques in and around brain cells.[19] However, recent studies have shown that declining acidity levels in lysosomes can lead to neurological damage associated with brain shrinkage.

A lysosome is an acidic type of membrane-bound organelle that contains digestive enzymes. Membrane-bound organelles are cellular structures bound by a biological membrane, which may be a single or double layer of lipids, typically with scattered

INTERMITTENT FASTING PLANS

Here are a few of the most common eight-hour eating windows:

9 a.m. to 5 p.m.	Have your first meal at 9 a.m. and finish your last meal by 5 p.m. This allows you to fast from 5 p.m. to 9 a.m. the following day, incorporating your sleep hours into the fasting period.
10 a.m. to 6 p.m.	You can eat between 10 a.m. and 6 p.m. and fast from 6 p.m. to 10 a.m. the next day.
12 p.m. to 8 p.m.	Opting for a 12-to-8 p.m. eating window results in a fasting interval from 8 p.m. to noon the next day, with the advantage of incorporating your overnight rest.

or interspersed proteins. Lysosomes have various cell functions, such as breaking down excess or worn-out cell parts. They can destroy invading viruses and bacteria and help damaged or dying cells to self-destruct in a process called programmed cell death or apoptosis. The acidic enzymes in lysosomes break down, remove, and recycle waste products such as excess plaque.

If you cannot live without breakfast, eat your food earlier in the day. If you can't imagine skipping dinner, eat your first meal a little later in the day (10 a.m. to 6 p.m.).

Sometimes the 16:8 diet is too much to take on, especially when one is facing a health crisis. In that case, there are other types of intermittent fasting you can try after discussing with your physician:

- *Alternate-day fasting.* Alternating between fasting days, during which you consume very few or no calories, and regular eating days.
- *5:2 diet.* Eating normally for five days a week and significantly reducing your calorie intake (to around 500–600 calories) on two non-consecutive days.
- *Eat-stop-eat.* Fasting for a full twenty-four hours once or twice a week.
- *The Warrior Diet.* Fasting for twenty hours each day and eating one large meal during the remaining four-hour window.

Some research has discovered that a drop in lysosome acidity levels may be a hidden culprit responsible for the onset of Alzheimer's disease.[20] While a slow buildup of beta-amyloid and tau proteins can cause plaques to manifest in and around brain cells, dysfunctional lysosomes may enhance that process, leading to neuronal damage. As a result, experimental therapy used to remove amyloid plaques has been largely unsuccessful in trying to halt the progression of the disease. Scientists are now working to develop treatments that target lysosome dysfunction and restore acidity levels.

While they do, there are actions you can take to boost lysosome function, particularly exercise and intermittent fasting.

FOODS THAT HAVE BEEN SHOWN TO HELP PREVENT ALZHEIMER'S DISEASE

- Beans and legumes
- Berries
- Fish
- Leafy green vegetables
- Nuts
- Olive oil
- Poultry
- Whole grains

THINGS YOU CAN DO FOR YOUR GUT AFTER AN ALZHEIMER'S DIAGNOSIS

- Consume pre- and probiotics every single day in addition to the nutrients you need (preferably as food, but in supplement form if necessary)
- Consider intermittent fasting
- Exercise

The latter is where the connection to the gut comes in, since what we put in our mouths travels through our gut and can end up impacting our brain. Early animal studies have shown some promise that fasting may delay the onset of vascular dementia and Alzheimer's disease and reduce brain inflammation.[21]

THE FIVE PILLARS AND CHANGING THE COURSE OF ALZHEIMER'S DISEASE

To date, the most common treatments for Alzheimer's disease have been medication and psychological support. But most drugs have proven effective only in improving symptoms, not in treating the cause of the disease. As noted earlier, the FDA has approved only a few drugs for the treatment of Alzheimer's. One of them, aducanumab, which targets beta-amyloid, works most effectively early in the course of the disease, and it is uncertain how much it helps in moderate and advanced cases. Medication is only one piece of the puzzle, however. What is missing in standard Alzheimer's care is treatment of the gut, something I believe will change as new research findings come in.

When it comes to the Five Pillars, we know how important nutrition is in changing the course of Alzheimer's, but another important pillar is movement (exercise). We have seen that exercise is beneficial for the gut and the brain, and this is especially the case when it comes to Alzheimer's disease. A thirty-five-year longitudinal study of over 2,000 men ages forty-five to fifty-nine years in Wales assessed five behaviors—smoking, alcohol intake, body weight, diet, and exercise—in relation to incidences of diabetes, vascular disease, cancer, death, and cognitive problems.

This data determined exercise had the greatest effect in terms of reducing dementia risk—by up to 60 percent.[22]

So do not neglect exercise in combination with nutrition, purpose, community, and spirituality as you become your own health hero and change the course of Alzheimer's disease.

CHAPTER EIGHT

HOW GUT HEALTH CONTRIBUTES TO PARKINSON'S DISEASE

Parkinson's disease (PD), the second-most-common neurodegenerative disorder, is primarily a disruption of the substantia nigra—a specific area of the brain where dopamine is produced. When this neurochemical imbalance occurs, systems of the central nervous system—like movement control, executive function, and behavior control—are impacted. Parkinson's is marked by tremors at rest, slowness of movement, and problems walking. Someone who has Parkinson's can look like they are slowing down, as if they just do not have much energy, or as if they're weak—symptoms typically associated with aging—so you might think that it is an older person's disease, but it can affect younger people as well. My friend Jimmy is a perfect example.

In our twenties, most of us are thriving and looking forward to building our lives and careers. Jimmy was the same, so when he started to notice minor physical changes, he brushed them off. He was busy living life—in his mid twenties he met a wonderful woman, and when they got married, his dad gave him some fatherly advice and suggested he buy life insurance. That is exactly what Jimmy did. During the life insurance exam, however, the nurse, who also happened to work in a neurologist's office, started asking him unexpected questions, like:

- Are you having trouble with your handwriting? Is it getting smaller?
- Has anyone commented that you speak quite softly and slur your words?
- Have people pointed out that you do not swing an arm when walking?
- Is constipation an issue for you?

When Jimmy answered yes to these and several more questions, she told him he needed to see a doctor as soon as possible. He did, and it turned out he had Parkinson's disease.

At first, Jimmy tried to ignore his diagnosis—he was only twenty-seven. But later, when he fell down a flight of stairs with his ten-month-old son in his arms, he heeded the wake-up call. Jimmy told me, "Everybody has to have that rock-bottom moment, and that was it for me. I realized I was becoming a danger to my kids and could become a burden instead of helping my wife raise our family."

As you will see in Chapter 9, by accepting and working with their disease and paying attention to the gut-brain connection, people like Jimmy may be able to turn their lives around.

MAJOR SYMPTOMS OF PARKINSON'S DISEASE

- *Cramping.* Twisting or tightening of one's muscles.
- *Drooling.* Compromised motor symptoms can lead to difficulty swallowing, excessive saliva, or drooling.
- *Dyskinesia.* Involuntary and erratic facial, trunk, leg, and arm movements.
- *Festination.* Short and rapid steps while walking, leading to frequent falls.
- *Freezing.* Parkinson's can lead to what seems like getting stuck in place during movement, which can increase the risk of falling.
- *Impaired balance and posture.*
- *Rigid muscles.* Stiffness that limits the range of motion and leads to pain.
- *Shuffling gait.* Short steps and a stooped posture.
- *Slowed movement.* Slowed movement (bradykinesia) and reduced ability to perform movement-related tasks, including walking, dressing, or getting out of a chair.
- *Masked face.* Slowed movement and rigidity can lead to an expressionless appearance.
- *Speech changes.* Speech may become soft, slurred, quick, hesitant, or monotone.
- *Tremor.* Shaking; often starts in a limb, especially the fingers or hand.
- *Writing changes.* Parkinson's may make writing difficult or lead to smaller handwriting.

WHAT IS PARKINSON'S DISEASE?

As with stroke and Alzheimer's disease, patients who present with Parkinson's are often like Jimmy: they tend to look healthy, at least until complications like uncontrollable tremors and even depression and bladder dysfunction rob them of a full life, often for decades.

Parkinson's is fairly common, affecting up to 2 percent of people over the age of sixty, but, as with Jimmy, it can strike at any age. Up to 80 percent of people with Parkinson's will develop dementia during the course of the disease.[1] Exposure to certain toxins or environmental factors can increase risk at a small level. Head injuries, age, gender, residence (living close to environmental toxins), and occupation (intensive physical labor and working with toxins) may also increase the risks of Parkinson's.

Parkinson's disease can be very subtle. Someone who has Parkinson's can feel like they are slowing down, like they just do not have much energy, or as though they are just weak. Parkinson's is a disorder of the brain. It occurs when the dopamine-producing

WHO IS AT RISK FOR PARKINSON'S DISEASE?

- *Age and gender.* Parkinson's disease affects 2 million Americans and 10 million people worldwide and is more common among people over sixty, especially men.[2]

- *Genes.* The exact reason Parkinson's occurs is unknown, but genes and the environment can play a role in its development. Certain uncommon genetic variants can lead to Parkinson's disease in rare cases, so pay attention if your family members have been affected by the disease, as genetic testing is not yet readily available.
- *External triggers.* Exposure to certain toxins or environmental elements can add to the risk of Parkinson's, so residence (living close to environmental toxins), and occupation (intensive physical labor or working with toxins) may increase the risks of Parkinson's. Head injuries can also be a factor.
- *Changes in the brain.* Certain changes in the brain can occur in people with Parkinson's disease, but why and when these happen is currently unknown. One of these changes is the presence of Lewy bodies in the brain cells, and also the alpha-synuclein proteins found in these Lewy bodies.[3]
- *Consuming animal products.* Those who already have certain risk factors, like advanced age and particularly an epigenetic predisposition, may increase their likelihood of initiating the disease by consuming animal products (meat and perhaps milk) that contain α-synuclein, which may escape the gut and cross the blood-brain barrier.[4]

cells in the substantia nigra are lost, leading to symptoms like tremors at rest, slowness of movement, and gait problems. To better understand Parkinson's, we need to understand Lewy bodies, which most people with Parkinson's (except for the small subset whose condition is the result of a specific genetic variant) have in their brain.

UNDERSTANDING LEWY BODIES

In Parkinson's disease, the genes responsible for the production of alpha-synuclein—a neuronal protein that regulates synaptic vesicle trafficking and subsequent neurotransmitter release—are overexpressed, and so the protein accumulates. These neuronal proteins combine to create something called Lewy bodies, which are clumps of abnormal proteins that are toxic to the brain. Specifically, Lewy bodies kill nerve cells in the brain responsible for producing dopamine, a neurotransmitter responsible for feelings of pleasure and motivation. Dopamine also sends messages to the part of the brain that controls movement, which is why people with Parkinson's disease who are lacking adequate levels of this neurotransmitter lose their sense of balance, become uncoordinated, and shake uncontrollably. These clusters can also lead to memory or cognitive problems, visual hallucinations, and difficulties with alertness.[5]

We do not fully understand why Lewy bodies accumulate in the brain, but their presence is undeniably considered to be the hallmark of Parkinson's. As we'll see, new research is showing that the source of Lewy bodies may actually begin in none other than the gut. Scientists are discussing this research in their debate about the origin of Parkinson's disease.[6] Dysbiosis, or an imbalance in the gut microbiome, can trigger the alpha-synuclein clusters that form Lewy bodies.

THE GUT-FIRST HYPOTHESIS

In a person with leaky gut or intestinal permeability, Lewy bodies can make their way into the second brain—the gut's enteric nervous system.[7] They travel via the gut-brain axis up into the "first" brain, where they begin their work of destroying neuronal cells. In response to this cell death, several other processes occur that reduce the amount of short-chain fatty acids that defend

COMPLICATIONS OF PARKINSON'S DISEASE

- Bladder problems
- Blood pressure changes
- Constipation
- Depression
- Emotional changes
- Fatigue
- Pain
- Problems swallowing
- Sexual dysfunction
- Sleep problems
- Smell dysfunction
- Thinking difficulties

and protect the central nervous system, allowing immune cells to blast through the blood-brain barrier, causing inflammation within the brain and creating an environment ripe for Parkinson's disease as well as other brain attacks.[8]

Evidence is beginning to suggest that gut disturbances precede Parkinson's neurological symptoms, sometimes by years. Rebecca was a longtime patient who suffered from intermittent constipation, bloating, and occasional trouble swallowing. During one appointment, she told me that after noticing a persistent tremor, she had been diagnosed with Parkinson's. She was early in her diagnosis of Parkinson's and was being treated by her neurologist.

I was sorry to hear it, but not surprised. Many patients suffering from Parkinson's display gastrointestinal symptoms. There is a current debate among scientists as to whether, after taking into account age, environment, and genetics, the origins of Parkinson's disease lie in the gut or the brain. As I mentioned, evidence is growing for a "gut-first" hypothesis, suggesting that the genesis of the disease is in the abnormal alpha-synuclein proteins escaping the gut and affecting the enteric nervous system. (This points to why constipation is considered a risk factor, since it affects up to two-thirds of Parkinson's patients.[9]) Other GI disorders (including infections, microbial imbalance, inflammation, and irritable bowel syndrome) as well as dietary factors have been linked to Parkinson's onset and progression, and have been shown to influence the response to PD medication.[10] If we can be proactive, then we may have a chance to intervene with patients like Rebecca to potentially ward off future problems with Parkinson's.

PEOPLE WITH PARKINSON'S ARE PRONE TO CONSTIPATION (AND POSSIBLY VICE VERSA)

As I noted above, one of Rebecca's symptoms was of particular interest to me: constipation. This is not to say that constipation causes or is even necessarily a sign of Parkinson's disease, but there certainly are some compelling correlations. Current research has shown us that constipation is one of Parkinson's most common GI features, affecting over 50 percent of all patients at some point during the course of their disease.[11] More important, constipation is now seen as a crucial prodromal symptom, appearing sometimes decades before the more readily diagnosed symptoms of Parkinson's, such as problems with gait, motion, speech, and balance.

This means the occurrence and acuteness of constipation in Parkinson's disease tends to correspond with the course of the disease, especially the issues of movement as well as cognitive decline and even depression. This is likely a consequence of the effect of the diseased brain on one or some of the muscle groups that help us defecate, such as the rectum and anal sphincter.[12]

DIETARY FACTORS

What we put into our mouths impacts our gut and consequently our brain. Recent studies have shown time and again that there is a correlation between certain foods and Parkinson's disease.[13] Researchers from Purdue University's School of Health Sciences have provided particular clarification. They have found a variety of dietary factors connected to Parkinson's disease, focusing on fats, vitamins, antioxidants, and minerals, as well as pesticides. People with optimal intakes of vitamin A and carotenoids, B vitamins and folates, and vitamin D tend to have a lower risk of Parkinson's disease, so one can hypothesize that the converse is true—low dietary levels or deficiencies of these nutrients could influence the likelihood of presenting with the disease. Foods containing magnesium showed a protective effect against Parkinson's disease.[14]

People who have a healthy intake of vitamin E, which can be found in vegetable oils, nuts, and whole-grain products, especially tend to have a lower incidence of Parkinson's. In part this may be because of the overlap between foods with vitamin E and foods that provide some omega-3 fatty acids. People who consume a healthy amount of omega-3 fatty acids (found in foods like oily fish, flaxseeds, chia seeds, and walnuts) have a lower risk of Parkinson's. This is because omega-3 deficiency affects the pathway by which dopamine travels in the brain, which is directly relevant to Parkinson's. However, a higher intake of animal fats has been linked with an increased risk of the disease, although further research is necessary.[15]

Exposure to pesticides has been consistently linked to Parkinson's. The pesticides rotenone and paraquat have been shown to induce dopaminergic neuron loss in the substantia nigra and corpus striatum in animals as well as in humans.[16] Such loss can lead to Parkinson's disease.[17] Some of the foods that are healthiest for our gut and our brain, and as a result are helpful in diminishing our risk for Parkinson's disease, are fruits (especially berries) and vegetables that, when produced conventionally, also tend to have higher concentrations of pesticides.

This is another reason it is especially important to eat organic whenever possible.

It is not just what we eat but how much. Studies have discovered that relatively low daily calorie intake (1,600–2,000 calories) beginning at approximately twenty years of age is likely to have a protective effect against Parkinson's.[18] So if you have a genetic predisposition to the disease, this is something you might want to pay attention to.

THE BIDIRECTIONAL APPROACH

Though, as we've seen, researchers who study the origins of Parkinson's are divided between those who promote a gut-first hypothesis and those who think a brain-first hypothesis is better, it is important to consider that the gut-brain axis is a two-way street—there is a bidirectional element. Many people with Parkinson's inherit the disease, so clearly gut health is not the only cause. However, it is becoming increasingly evident that the state of our gut is a key contributing factor that we have some agency over. We know that there is no reason for Lewy bodies to be present in the enteric nervous system, so by taking measures to improve gut health, we can prevent the environment that fosters Lewy body production.

We have also seen that GI disorders, including infections as well as microbial imbalance, inflammation, and irritable bowel syndrome, especially in combination with dietary factors, have been linked to Parkinson's onset and progression and have been shown to influence the effectiveness of PD medication.[19] The crux of the argument when it comes to Parkinson's and the gut is

WHAT YOU CAN DO FOR YOUR GUT TO PREVENT PARKINSON'S

- Pay attention to your genetic history, and if someone in your family has had Parkinson's, adjust your lifestyle accordingly, including limiting your consumption of animal products like meat and milk.
- If constipation is a problem for you, do not ignore it. Instead, address this by drinking plenty of water and by consuming fruit, fiber, and probiotics to improve bowel motility.
- Pay close attention to any signs that may be indicative of Parkinson's. Even if they are subtle, please ask your physician for guidance.
- Proactively avoid toxins in your home (such as dry-cleaning solvents) and work environments.[20] If your work involves the use of metal-degreasing chemicals, paint thinners, and strong detergents, take precautions, such as masking and ventilation.
- Reduce your exposure to pesticides by eating organic food wherever possible.
- Eat a balanced diet rich in fruits and vegetables, especially those containing vitamin A, B vitamins, and folate. Leafy greens, legumes, and broccoli are good choices. Not only will you help reduce your risk of Parkinson's, but you'll support your gut health and increase the diversity of your microbiome.

that there is good reason to think that the gut-brain connection can allow inflammation to occur in the brain, and when that happens, Parkinson's may become a reality.

As we have seen throughout this book, gut disturbances have been linked to brain disorders—not just Parkinson's but stroke and Alzheimer's. Although, as I noted earlier, the composition of the gut microbiota remains relatively stable once it is established at the end of adolescence, it is constantly affected by external factors such as environment, medication, nutrition, and exercise, which are things we can have an impact on. So there are actions we can take that may have a role in the possible intervention in and even prevention of brain disorders.[21]

CHAPTER NINE

CHANGING THE COURSE OF PARKINSON'S DISEASE

After accepting his Parkinson's disease diagnosis, Jimmy became a health hero. He completely turned his life around, embracing all Five Pillars. His purpose became being there for his family. As well as changing his diet, he started walking around the block each day to develop strength and stamina, which led to walking farther, improving his symptoms and ultimately his overall health. Little things added up, and over time he even started running marathons. When I last heard from him, he had completed more than fifteen marathons, had done more than a hundred half marathons, and had even appeared on *American Ninja Warrior*. He found community by inspiring others through his involvement with the Michael J. Fox Foundation for Parkinson's Research. Jimmy's message is, "Everybody is faced with some type of adversity. The idea is never to give up." With the ever-evolving ways we can change the course of Parkinson's through gut health and the Five Pillars, there is more hope than ever before.

LEWY BODIES AND GUT INTEGRITY

In the previous chapter I introduced Lewy bodies—the abnormal clusters of a neuronal protein called alpha-synuclein—that are toxic to the brain and directly linked to Parkinson's disease. Think about Lewy bodies like craters after a bombing. First, we need to try to find out what caused the destruction. Was it a plane? A tank? If it was a plane, how do we stop the plane from flying? If it is a tank, how do we stop it from rolling? Once we know the specific route the bombers are taking and the methods they are using, we can put into place obstacles to prevent their attack. In the case of Parkinson's, we do not always understand how the destruction began, because so many different things can lead to the disease. However, what we can do is eliminate factors that make it worse. Here, we can protect the enteric nervous system and perhaps help prevent the Lewy bodies from occurring in the brain.

Parkinson's has no known cure, and treatment for the disease does not slow or stop progression. Though researchers have known about this unrelenting neurodegenerative disorder for more than two centuries and have studied it extensively, the most common treatment that most doctors prescribe is levodopa, a medication used to try to increase dopamine levels and improve motor function. While it can be effective for a time, the treatment has significant neurological side effects and is no match for Parkinson's unrelenting pathophysiology. The Lewy bodies eventually decimate the patient's brain neurologically.[1]

Mainstream medicine also prescribes physical therapy, which I fully support. As we know from Jimmy's story, if started early enough after onset, exercise and physical therapy have been shown to slow or decrease Parkinson's effects.

To attack Parkinson's, we need to prevent the alpha-synuclein clusters from forming in the first place. The first goal is gut integrity, which we can achieve through a diet low in fat and high in fiber, as well as by prescribing selective probiotics based on an individual's microbiome profile. Improvements in Parkinson's are associated with microbes such as *Lactobacillus* and *Bifidobacterium* and with the postbiotic butyrate (see Chapter 7). In mice who have been given *Lactobacillus*, levels of interleukin-6 and tumor necrosis factor (TNF)—both known inflammatory substances—have been shown to decrease, improving motor deficits and relieving Parkinson's-associated constipation.[2] Although the diagnostics used to measure the composition of the gut microbiome have not been standardized and are not guaranteed to be 100 percent accurate, taking these pro- and postbiotics aims to prevent and to heal.

If Parkinson's is present in members of the patient's family, we must be even more vigilant since there is a hereditary component to this disease. I recommend using the Five Pillars as a preventive measure. Even if the disease process has begun, in many instances nutrition, movement, purpose, community, and spirituality in concert can slow decline and improve symptoms, as we have seen.

WHAT STARTS IN THE GUT ENDS UP IN THE BRAIN (AND BEYOND)

Information is accumulating about how Parkinson's disease may start in the gut and travel to the brain. To explore how the microbiome plays into this, neurologists from the University of Alabama and their colleagues conducted a large-scale study of 490 people with Parkinson's and 234 control subjects.[3] They analyzed fecal DNA, looking to identify potentially infectious and disease-indicating polymicrobial clusters. "The primary aim of this study was to generate a full, unaltered view of the dysbiosis in PD gut microbiome."

They found that 30 percent of these polymicrobial species that were studied had Parkinson's disease, constituting an extensive dysbiosis in the microbiome. They further observed that the Parkinson's-associated clusters grow together, showing that the Parkinson's microbiome may be "disease permissive"—that is, it can create an ecosystem where the conditions for the disease flourish. The researchers concluded by saying, "We uncovered a widespread dysbiosis in PD metagenome that is indicative of an environment permissive for neurodegenerative events and prohibitive of recovery."[4] They offered hope that the tools and analytical techniques they used in this study will help researchers look more deeply at the origin and progression of Parkinson's, identify biomarkers, and "investigate the potential in manipulating the microbiome to prevent, treat and halt the progression of PD."[5] In other words, scientists are once again demonstrating that what starts in the gut ends up in the brain . . . and it affects the rest of our bodies as well.

Current and ongoing investigations into the microbiome and Parkinson's disease are finding patterns when it comes to tremors—one of the most common outward symptoms of Parkinson's disease. When researchers investigated the gut microbiota composition in Parkinson's patients in relation to how pronounced their tremors were, by analyzing fecal samples, they found a reduction in the relative abundance of certain bacteria (those in the genera *Blautia, Coprococcus,* and *Lachnospira*) and an increase in other bacteria (in the genera *Escherichia* and *Serratia*) in those who exhibited fewer tremors. Likewise, the levels of important molecules (i.e., nicotinic acid, cadaverine, and glucuronic acid) varied in relation to the severity of symptoms.[6] This raises the possibility that introducing specific bacteria into the gut through fecal transplants or pre- and probiotics may not only impact the progression of the disease but also decrease one of its most debilitating manifestations: tremors.

PREBIOTICS, PROBIOTICS, AND POSTBIOTICS

I saw the results of this manner of addressing gut issues in a powerful way while working with my patient Vivian. She was a wonderful woman—a community leader, a devoted mother and wife. I met her after she was diagnosed with Parkinson's disease and was managing it with medications and courses of physical therapy; however, the disease was progressing. Vivian was referred to me for a colonoscopy after symptoms of bloating and constipation. I gave her pre- and probiotics as well as post-biotics to nourish her microbiome and support her gut health.

Essentially, postbiotics can be defined as the substances microorganisms produce or leave behind that have a positive effect on our gut health. Some postbiotics slow the growth of harmful bacteria; others, such as the SCFA butyrate, help healthy bacteria flourish. Among other things, postbiotics support the immune system and reduce inflammation, allowing the GI barrier to retain or repair its integrity.

Not only did this course of pre-, pro-, and postbiotic treatment significantly improve Vivian's gastrointestinal symptoms, but something remarkable happened when we introduced these new organisms into her microbiome: her Parkinson's symptoms

SOURCES OF POSTBIOTICS

- Blue cheese
- Kefir
- Kimchi
- Kombucha
- Natto (fermented soybean paste)
- Pickled vegetables
- Sauerkraut
- Swiss cheese
- Tempeh
- Vinegar
- Yogurt

also improved. It was fantastic for Vivian to experience how gut health can improve brain health, as it added quality to her life and eased her decline.

Physicians are increasingly interested in the power of postbiotics to treat Parkinson's disease. Although more research is necessary to determine exactly what is responsible for their positive effects, this is likely because of their immunomodulatory

FOODS THAT POSITIVELY IMPACT PARKINSON'S DISEASE

As well as pre-, pro-, and postbiotics, other foods have been shown to correlate with decreasing the symptoms of Parkinson's disease.[7] Adding nutrition-dense, fresh, organic whole foods, such as greens, other vegetables and fruits, can be beneficial for people with Parkinson's. And a diet high in fiber and low in processed carbs and bad fats can help in prevention as well.[8]

- *Raw foods.* Raw green vegetables are high in antioxidants and can fight inflammation and pain in the body.
- *High-fiber foods.* Foods rich in fiber can help with bowel function, which can be a problem for those with Parkinson's.
- *Healthy fats.* Healthy fats, such as those found in avocados, coconuts, nuts, seeds, and wild-caught

(influencing the immune system by boosting or calming its activity), anti-inflammatory, anti-obesogenic (interfering with fat storage), anti-proliferative (slowing uncontrolled growth of cells), anti-hypertensive, hypocholesterolemic (lowering cholesterol levels), and antioxidant capabilities. Among these post-biotics, SCFAs in particular were found to be especially valuable. Animal studies have shown that SCFA butyrate can improve

fish, can improve brain and neurological functions, as well as mood.

- *Cold-pressed oils.* Cold-pressed oils are rich in essential vitamin E and can reduce inflammation.
- *Omega-3.* Omega-3 supplements and foods rich in omega-3s, such as wild seafood, algae, seeds, and nuts, can boost dopamine levels and improve inflammation.
- *Fresh vegetable juices.* Green juices in particular can help with hydration and constipation.
- *Moderate protein intake.* Keeping protein intake low to moderate can improve symptoms.
- *Olives.* Researchers are finding that a compound present in olives called hydroxytyrosol helps support dopamine levels and may significantly ease Parkinson's motor symptoms.[9]
- *Brewed tea.* Higher consumption of brewed tea has been associated with a lower risk of Parkinson's disease.[10]

Parkinson's-related motor damage and dopamine deficiency, as well as slowing or decreasing neuroinflammation.[11]

COFFEE, TEA, AND CONSTIPATION

We saw in Chapter 8 that there is a connection between Parkinson's disease and constipation. Several studies have shown that people who consume caffeinated beverages such as coffee, tea (especially black tea), and even energy drinks, sodas, and chocolate tend to have a decreased risk of Parkinson's disease.[12] This is in part because caffeine stimulates the central nervous system and is known to be an adenosine receptor antagonist, which means it binds to adenosine receptors and affects various

REMOVE FOODS THAT CAN MAKE PARKINSON'S SYMPTOMS WORSE

Reducing the amount of these foods in the diet, or eliminating them altogether, can help alleviate the symptoms of Parkinson's.

- *Excessive animal protein.* Ideally, aim for 0.36 grams of protein per day per pound of body weight.
- *Highly processed foods.*
- *Refined sugar and artificial sweeteners.*
- *Alcohol.*
- *Any potential food allergens and foods to which you may be sensitive.*[13]

bodily functions including sleep, blood flow, and breathing. Not only might caffeine have a neuroprotective effect, but it also can have positive effects on both cognitive and motor abilities. This is because caffeine provides neuroprotection against dopaminergic neurodegeneration since "Caffeine's action is largely mediated by the brain adenosine A2A receptor (A2AR) and confer neuro-protection by modulating neuroinflammation and excitotoxicity and mitochondrial function."[14]

MEAT, DAIRY, AND PARKINSON'S DISEASE

Recent dietary studies have shown a connection between consuming animal products and the risk of Parkinson's disease.[15] Evidence has been found that a particular heterocyclic amine—one of a number of toxic carcinogenic and mutagenic chemicals that form when muscle meats such as beef, pork, fowl, and fish are cooked at high temperatures—is elevated in the brains of Parkinson's disease patients.[16] Likewise, there's an association between higher consumption of animal fats and a higher risk of Parkinson's disease even twenty to thirty years before the clinical onset of the disease. This can be as much as two to nine times higher, although a causal effect hasn't been fully proven.[17]

Meat is not the only culprit. Consumption of dairy prod-ucts has been associated with escalation of the probability of Parkinson's disease, particularly in men, although more study is necessary.[18]

When it comes to risk factors, since many people eat meat and consume dairy products but only a small percentage of them develop Parkinson's disease, it is more likely that this is a contributing factor in concert with aging, a genetic and/or epigenetic predisposition, and inflammation creating an environment for Parkinson's disease to develop.

THE GLYMPHATIC SYSTEM AND SLEEPING ON THE SIDE

Another unusual connection to Parkinson's disease has been observed in how we sleep. It turns out that sleeping on your side improves the glymphatic system, the network of systems that plays a vital role in removing waste and toxins from the brain.[19] To grasp the gut-brain benefits of sleeping on your side, especially when it comes to changing the course of neurodegenerative diseases like Parkinson's, it is essential to understand the glymphatic system—which plays a vital role in removing waste and toxins from the brain. It operates most actively during sleep, and research has shown that it is crucial for maintaining brain health. The importance of this system is especially relevant considering that problems with gut health may be the reason you cannot sleep.

Scientific studies have revealed that sleeping on your side can enhance the function of the glymphatic system, facilitating more efficient removal of waste and toxins from the brain. In a study published in the *Journal of Neuroscience*, researchers found that sleeping on the side in general increased cerebrospinal fluid transport through the glymphatic system, and thus could potentially lead to improved brain health.[20] Furthermore, this study suggests that sleeping on the side may reduce the risk of developing neurological conditions such as Alzheimer's disease and Parkinson's disease.

In addition to its impact on brain health, sleeping on the side can also benefit your stomach and consequently the gut as a whole. This position allows the stomach to rest below the esophagus, which can help prevent acid reflux and heartburn.

OPTIMIZING SLEEPING ON YOUR SIDE

- *Use a supportive pillow.* Select a pillow that provides adequate support to ensure proper alignment of your head, neck, and spine.
- *Keep your legs slightly bent.* To prevent lower back pain, maintain a slight bend in your legs while sleeping on your side.
- *Experiment with various positions.* While sleeping on the side offers numerous benefits, it is crucial to find the sleeping position that works best for you and your body. Some individuals may find variations, such as a slight tilt or additional pillows, more comfortable and equally beneficial.
- *Transition gradually.* If you are accustomed to sleeping on your back, transitioning to sleeping on your side may take time. Gradually introduce this position by using pillows to support your body and prevent rolling onto your back. Loose-fitting clothing can also aid in the transition and minimize discomfort.

A study published in the *Journal of Clinical Gastroenterology* investigated the effect of sleep position on gastroesophageal reflux disease. The researchers found that sleeping on your side can significantly reduce the occurrence of acid reflux episodes compared to other positions, providing empirical evidence for the benefits of this sleep posture.[21]

WALKING MEDITATION AND THE GUT-BRAIN AXIS

Walking meditation has been shown to have an impact on functional performance, disease severity, and anxiety in patients with Parkinson's disease.[22] Although methods may vary, a simple and sustainable walking meditation is related to the Zen practice of *kinhin.* Here is how to do it.

- Find a location to walk without distractions. It should be a peaceful place. Make sure the path you have chosen is fairly easy and you have any physical support you might need, so that you can focus on just walking, not navigation.
- Lower your gaze, but do not be inattentive, especially when walking outdoors.
- Become conscious of your breath (but do not try to control it) as you begin walking slowly—very slowly—and deliberately. Notice the rise and fall of your chest and the feeling of the air as it enters and leaves your lungs.

Moreover, sleeping on your side promotes healthy digestion. By positioning the body this way, food can move more easily through your intestines, aiding in regular bowel movements and preventing constipation, which is particularly an issue in Parkinson's disease.

- Feel the entire motion of your footfall, from heel touching ground to toe rising, as your weight shifts. Then the next step, and the next.
- Your pace should be slow enough that you can remain aware of each step and breath. Now, move even more slowly.
- Be aware of your body. As you walk, pay attention to your posture and your body's alignment. Keep your back straight and your shoulders relaxed. All the while, notice the sensations in your feet as they contact the ground and your breath in unison.
- Let go of thoughts. Use the process of walking and breathing to keep you connected to the present moment.
- Be compassionate and patient with yourself. Your mind will wander, and when it does, gently bring it back to your breath or your body.
- There is no set minimum or maximum time for walking meditation. You can practice for as long as you like.[23]

CENTERING PRAYER

Another piece of the spirituality pillar is prayer. Interestingly, centering prayer may have an impact on Parkinson's disease. Researchers anecdotally noticed symptom reduction in a patient who practiced centering prayer, which led them to study a small group of people with Parkinson's disease before and after practicing.[24] They assessed tremors via electromyography (EMG) and found that patients showed a significant reduction in EMG amplitude after a centering prayer session.

Although this important insight deserves further research, centering prayer is a simple and accessible practice:

- Select a word or symbol that is meaningful or sacred to you.
- Sit in a comfortable position, close your eyes, and settle your body and breath.
- Silently hold your sacred word or symbol in your mind.
- As your thoughts drift, gently return to your sacred word or symbol.
- As you complete the practice, sit in silence with your eyes closed for a few moments.

THE FIVE PILLARS AND CHANGING THE COURSE OF PARKINSON'S DISEASE

Vivian's experience showed us how applying the Five Pillars can influence the course of Parkinson's disease, and especially the effect that nutrition can have. And as we saw with Jimmy, exercise can significantly slow progress of the disease, reducing

THINGS TO DO FOR YOUR GUT AFTER A PARKINSON'S DIAGNOSIS

- Eat less meat and more vegetables—especially cruciferous vegetables, like cauliflower, cabbage, kale, cress, bok choy, broccoli, and Brussels sprouts, which are rich in healthful substances, including glucoraphanin. This seems to help prevent the loss of dopamine and thus provide a potential preventative effect against Parkinson's disease.[25]
- Exercise within your capacities.
- Consume pre-, pro-, and postbiotics.
- While still controversial and not widely used, clinical trials show that fecal transplant—a procedure where feces are collected from a healthy donor and introduced into a patient's gastrointestinal tract—may increase diversity of the intestinal microbiome, reducing constipation and improving gut transit and intestinal motility. It may even improve some motor and non-motor symptoms.[26]

risk and diminishing complications. This is in part because exercise lowers inflammation, which, as we know, benefits the gut as well as the brain. Furthermore, it improves mood and hence often makes it easier to embrace a sense of purpose.[27]

Another pillar to pay attention to when it comes to Parkinson's disease is spirituality. Practices like tai chi and yoga (which can be done in community) not only improve balance in Parkinson's patients, reducing their risk of falling, but also improve their state of mind.[28] Likewise, simple mindfulness meditation practices and even centering prayer have been shown to decrease disease severity.[29]

THE RECIPES

My dad was a Renaissance man. He was a world-renowned polymer chemist, a beautiful singer and poet, and an excellent chef. Babuni, as my sister and I affectionately called him, created culinary masterpieces with spices, his brain, and the stove. On each special occasion, our family eagerly awaited his creative, delicious cuisine. Vegetable, fish, and chicken dishes with tantalizing aromas excited our family's senses and filled our hearts with delight when we entered the kitchen.

My love for cooking came from both my parents. My father and mother involved my sister and me in the process of preparing meals, and we laughed, shared stories, and ate together—helping me put the Five Pillars into practice even before I had names for them. Ours was a magical household, thanks in large part to our time in the family kitchen. I have tried to re-create this in my home, where my wife, our children, and I cook together, laughing and enjoying the community and spiritual connection we forge.

I want to extend this feeling of love and community in the following chapters, which are devoted to original recipes—some of which have been passed down from my family—that not only are gut-healthy in general but also, I now believe, can help

HERBS AND SPICES

If you are unfamiliar with some of the herbs or spices in these recipes, here are some reliable sources.

- Kalustyan's   www.foodsofnations.com
- Penzey's   www.penzeys.com
- Spicewalla   www.spicewallabrand.com

Many health food, grocery, and even big box stores now carry a wider selection of spices as well. No matter where you get your ingredients, be sure to make freshness, non-GMO production, and known organic sources a priority.

prevent each of the three neurodegenerative disorders covered in the book: stroke, Alzheimer's, and Parkinson's diseases. For each recipe, I note how the ingredients work to slow or prevent the development of the condition.

CHAPTER TEN

RECIPES TO HELP CHANGE THE COURSE OF STROKE

To prevent stroke, I recommend a well-balanced diet that not only fosters optimal gut health but also helps to control hypertension and diabetes, which are important risk factors. Sweet and white potatoes (with their skins), bananas, tomatoes, prunes, melon, and soybeans help control hypertension. Ginger is believed to have the potential to help prevent diabetes.[1] In addition, I favor foods high in magnesium, such as spinach, because the mineral has been shown to decrease the risk of stroke.

BANANA GINGER SMOOTHIE

Every ingredient in this recipe contributes to gut or heart health. Bananas are high in potassium, which supports healthy blood pressure, and that correlates with decreased incidence of stroke. Yogurt is an excellent probiotic, helping to populate the gut with beneficial bacteria. Raw honey is a prebiotic. (Be sure to look for labels that say "raw" and preferably "unfiltered," and avoid heating the honey, as it will lose its prebiotic properties if it reaches a temperature much greater than 95 degrees Fahrenheit.) Ginger has been cultivated as a healthful food in India and China for over 5,000 years and now is easily available worldwide.

Servings: 1

Ingredients

1 banana, sliced (and frozen if you wish)

6 ounces vanilla yogurt

1 tablespoon raw honey

½ teaspoon freshly grated ginger

Directions

1. Combine banana, yogurt, honey, and ginger in a blender.
2. Blend until smooth.
3. Drink at once.

RED CABBAGE AND SPINACH SALAD

This refreshing and easy salad is full of nutrients to enhance gut health and counteract stroke. Balsamic vinegar has been shown to help lower LDL cholesterol, as has cilantro.[2] Spinach is rich in potassium. Red cabbage is an often-neglected super-food packed with antioxidants and flavonoids including antho-cyanins, which studies have shown can protect and repair our blood-brain barrier.[3]

Servings: 4

Ingredients

½ cup orange juice

3 tablespoons balsamic vinegar

2 tablespoons honey or applesauce

¼ teaspoon salt

Dash of black pepper

4 cups thinly sliced red cabbage

½ pound baby spinach

2 large green onions, thinly sliced

1 tablespoon chopped cilantro

Directions

1. In a large bowl whisk together the orange juice, vinegar, honey or applesauce, salt, and pepper.
2. Arrange the cabbage in the center of a large serving platter. Place the spinach around the cabbage.
3. Sprinkle sliced green onion over the cabbage and spinach.
4. Drizzle about one-third of the dressing over the salad.
5. Top with cilantro.
6. Serve remaining dressing with the salad.

BUTTERNUT TIKKA MASALA

A family favorite, especially on a cold day, this vegetarian dish not only is delicious fresh from the stove but freezes and reheats quite well. Serve with brown or black rice as a main dish for a complete meal. The curcumin in turmeric has been shown to potentially delay the onset of stroke and increase survival time.[4]

Butternut squash is high in potassium, the tomatoes rich in flavo-noids. Beans in general are a heart-healthy food, and chickpeas in particular have been shown to contain gut bacterial metabolites that seem to contribute to post-stroke recovery.[5]

Servings: 4

Ingredients

> 6 cups butternut squash, peeled and cut into 1-inch cubes (one large or two small squash)
>
> 3 cups cooked chickpeas
>
> 4 tablespoons avocado oil
>
> ¾ teaspoon salt
>
> 2½ teaspoons garam masala spice blend (see page 187)
>
> ⅓ cup roughly chopped cilantro
>
> Yogurt (optional)

Sauce

½ cup peeled and sliced fresh ginger

15 cloves garlic, peeled

3 serrano chiles, cut lengthwise

6 tablespoons avocado oil

6 tablespoons tomato paste

2 teaspoons garam masala spice blend (see page 187)

1 teaspoon cinnamon

10 Roma tomatoes, roughly chopped

2 teaspoons salt

¾ teaspoon pepper

2½ cups water

1½ cans (about 18 ounces) coconut milk

GARAM MASALA SPICE BLEND

This works well with pre-ground spices, but if you have the time to toast and pulverize whole coriander seed, cumin seed, cloves, and cardamom pods, it will enhance the flavor and add nutrients. Garam masala can add flavor and nutrients to curries, stews, soups, marinades, and even cookies or cakes.

Makes about ⅓ cup

Ingredients
- 4 teaspoons ground cumin
- 4 teaspoons ground coriander
- 4 teaspoons ground cinnamon
- 2 teaspoons ground cardamom
- 2 teaspoons ground cloves

Directions
1. Combine spices in a small bowl and mix well.
2. Store in an airtight container.

Directions
1. Preheat oven to 400° Fahrenheit.
2. In a large mixing bowl, combine squash, chickpeas, 4 tablespoons avocado oil, salt, and garam masala. Toss well.
3. Spread the squash mixture on a parchment-lined pan and bake 30–35 minutes, stirring several times.

4. Meanwhile, make the sauce. In a food processor, combine ginger, garlic, and serrano chiles. Pulse until finely chopped.

5. Heat 6 tablespoons of avocado oil in a large pot over medium heat.

6. Add ginger mixture and sauté 8–9 minutes until golden, stirring frequently and scraping the pan to make sure nothing sticks.

7. Add the tomato paste and cook 3–4 minutes.

8. Add garam masala and cinnamon. Cook 1–2 minutes.

9. Add tomatoes, salt, pepper, and water. Bring to a boil, then reduce the heat to low and simmer 20–22 minutes. Remove from heat and allow to cool for a few minutes.

10. In a food processor, blend the sauce mixture in small batches until it reaches a fairly smooth texture.

11. Return the sauce mixture to the pot, add coconut milk, and whisk well.

12. Add the roasted squash mixture and simmer 8–10 minutes.

13. Garnish with cilantro and a dollop of yogurt, if desired.

LENTIL STEW WITH SPINACH AND POTATOES

Legumes, including lentils, have been associated with a lower risk of cardiovascular disease and stroke.[6] Potato skins are rich in potassium and magnesium, and sweet potatoes are not only low on the glycemic index but also high in disease-fighting phytochemicals and antioxidants. Lemons are full of vitamin C; in addition, studies have found that ingesting fresh lemon juice can reduce stroke risk by up to 19 percent because the flavanones in lemons (and several other fruits) are believed to reduce oxidative stress and contribute to better blood flow to the brain.[7]

Servings: 4

Ingredients

> 2 tablespoons olive oil
>
> 2 large garlic cloves, chopped
>
> 3 cups fresh or canned vegetable broth (low sodium if possible)
>
> 1 cup lentils, rinsed and picked over
>
> 4 ounces (about ½ cup) red-skinned potatoes, cut into ½-inch pieces
>
> 4 ounces sweet potato, cut into ½-inch pieces
>
> 1 lemon
>
> 6 ounces fresh spinach, torn
>
> ¼ teaspoon cayenne
>
> ¼ cup chopped fresh mint
>
> Salt
>
> Black pepper
>
> Crumbled feta cheese (optional)

Directions

1. Heat oil in a heavy large saucepan over medium heat.
2. Add garlic and cook, stirring, 30 seconds.
3. Add vegetable broth and lentils. Bring to a boil, then reduce the heat and simmer, covered, for 10 minutes.

4. Add red-skinned and sweet potatoes. Cook, uncovered, stirring occasionally, until potatoes and lentils are tender, about 15 minutes.

5. Grate ½ teaspoon of peel from the lemon. Squeeze enough juice from the lemon to measure 2 tablespoons.

6. Add lemon peel, lemon juice, spinach, and cayenne to the lentil-potato mixture.

7. Cover and simmer until spinach wilts and is cooked through, about 2 minutes.

8. Mix in the mint.

9. Season with salt and pepper to taste.

10. Spoon stew into large soup bowls.

11. Sprinkle feta cheese over the dish, if desired.

CHAPTER ELEVEN

RECIPES TO HELP CHANGE THE COURSE OF ALZHEIMER'S DISEASE

When it comes to Alzheimer's disease, I recommend the Mediterranean diet, with an emphasis on plant-based ingredients. Foods high in saturated fat, such as red meat, should be consumed only occasionally, if at all. Simple and refined sugars should be avoided. Eat at least six servings of leafy green vegetables every week, along with organic (if possible) berries, whole grains, fish, poultry, beans, and nuts. Studies have shown that this food plan has been related to decreased cognitive decline and improved verbal memory, and it can reduce the risk of developing Alzheimer's disease.[1]

BRAIN-BOOSTING FISH FILLETS

Fish, especially wild-caught, is brain food. Haddock is a reliable source of omega-3 fatty acids and polyunsaturated fat (the same type of fat that our brain is made of). Avocado oil is heart healthy. It is a monounsaturated fat that helps to lower "bad" cholesterol. Garlic has many benefits, including antioxidant qualities, which can help prevent cognitive decline. How you season this dish is up to you—try it with garam masala, for an Indian take, or with Provençal herbs (thyme, basil, rosemary, tarragon, savory, marjoram, oregano, bay leaf) for a completely different yet equally delicious flavor profile.

Servings: 4

Ingredients

2 tablespoons avocado oil

6 garlic cloves, peeled and crushed

2 pints cherry tomatoes, halved

2 tablespoons dry white wine

Four 5-ounce haddock fillets

Your favorite seasoning blend (see recipe headnote for suggestions)

½ cup Kalamata olives, pitted

1 cup finely chopped fresh basil

Directions

1. Preheat the oven to 425° Fahrenheit.
2. Heat avocado oil in an oven-safe skillet over medium heat.
3. Add garlic and sauté for 1–2 minutes, or until fragrant, stirring frequently.
4. Add tomatoes to the skillet and stir.
5. Add white wine and stir well. Remove from heat.
6. Season fillets with your favorite seasoning blend.

7. Add fillets to the pan, making sure they are in contact with the pan surface.
8. Top fillets with olives and basil. Spoon some tomatoes and pan juices over the fillets.
9. Place in oven and bake for 10–15 minutes, until the fish is cooked through.

COCONUT CURRY CHICKEN

Curry powder includes so many spices that are good for our gut and our brain. Coconut oil is currently being studied for its potential to diminish the severity of Alzheimer's disease.[2] Nuts are sources of omega-3 fatty acids. You can substitute chickpeas and/or potatoes for the chicken and use vegetable broth to make this a vegetarian dish.

Servings: 4

Ingredients

    4 boneless, skinless chicken breasts, cut into strips
    1½ cups low-sodium chicken broth
    1½ cups coconut milk
    2 tablespoons curry powder (store-bought or homemade, see page 194)
    1 cup golden raisins
    1 cup unsalted peanuts or cashews (reserve half for garnish, if desired)
    2 cups cooked jasmine rice
    Salt

CURRY POWDER

Store-bought curry powders are convenient and tasty, especially if they have not been on the shelf for too long, but if
you would like to make your own, start with the whole spices
listed here. Here is the combination I like, but the beautiful
thing about making it yourself is you can adjust for your
palate and your tolerance for heat.

Makes about ½ cup

Ingredients
- 2–3 tablespoons black peppercorns
- ½ teaspoon shelled cardamom pods
- 2 dried hot chiles (like chile de árbol, chipotle, or ancho), seeds and stems removed
- 1-inch piece cinnamon stick
- ½ teaspoon whole cloves
- 2 tablespoons coriander seed
- 2 tablespoons cumin seed
- 1 teaspoon fennel seed
- 2 teaspoons fenugreek seeds
- 2–3 pieces long pepper (pippali), or 1 teaspoon Szechuan peppercorns
- 2 teaspoons mustard seeds
- 3 tablespoons ground dried turmeric
- 1 tablespoon ground dried ginger

Directions

1. Toast all the spices except for the turmeric and ginger in a dry pan over medium heat for 2–4 minutes. Let cool.
2. Grind or pulverize dry spices with a mortar and pestle or spice grinder until fine enough to sift through a sieve.
3. Mix in the ground turmeric and ginger.
4. Store in an airtight container.

Directions

1. Combine chicken, broth, coconut milk, curry powder, raisins, and nuts in a crockpot, turn on medium heat, and cook for approximately two hours.
2. Pour the cooked chicken mixture over the hot jasmine rice.
3. Season with salt to taste. (If you reserved half the nuts, garnish the dish with the remaining nuts.)

DR. NANDI'S BERRY DELICIOUS SALAD

Many recent studies show that regularly eating berries is associated with a reduced risk of Alzheimer's neuropathology.[3] Berries are high in pelargonidin, a bioactive compound rich in antioxidant and anti-inflammatory properties, as is spinach. Fermented dairy products like blue cheese and yogurt have preventive effects against dementia, and so do the "good" fats found in almonds and avocado. Even the basil in this easy-to-make salad serves a purpose, as it has a compound called fenchol, which may reduce damage in the Alzheimer's brain.[4]

Servings: 4

Ingredients

9 ounces baby spinach, torn

1 cup sliced strawberries

1 cup raspberries

1 cup blueberries

½ cup sliced almonds, toasted

⅓ cup chopped basil

1 avocado, chopped

4 ounces blue cheese

Strawberry or raspberry balsamic vinegar

Directions

1. Divide baby spinach among four plates.
2. Top with berries, almonds, basil, and chopped avocado.
3. Crumble blue cheese on top.
4. Drizzle with strawberry or raspberry balsamic vinegar to taste.

ALMOND NUTMEG COOKIES

These cookies are based on a traditional and beloved Indian treat called nankhatai and are full of brain-healthy spices and omega-rich nut oils. If you have access to besan (also called gram flour), be sure to use it, because this chickpea-based flour is high in both fiber and protein. If you don't, substitute additional whole-wheat or almond flour.

Servings: Makes 2 dozen cookies

Ingredients

- 1 cup all-purpose flour
- ½ cup whole-wheat flour
- ½ cup superfine almond flour
- ½ cup besan (or substitute additional whole-wheat or almond flour)
- 2 tablespoons semolina
- ¾ cup granulated sugar
- 2 teaspoons powdered cardamom (or 4–5 pods, crushed)
- ¼ teaspoon ground nutmeg (freshly grated if possible)
- 2 teaspoons baking powder
- 1 cup ghee or 8 ounces melted butter
- 2 tablespoons warm milk (if needed)
- ½ cup chopped almonds
- 2–4 tablespoons chopped pistachios, almonds, and dried cherries (for garnish)

Directions

1. Preheat the oven to 350° Fahrenheit.
2. Sift together the all-purpose flour, whole-wheat flour, almond flour, almonds, and besan. Add the semolina, sugar, cardamom, nutmeg, and baking powder and mix well.

3. Add the ghee or melted butter and mix until incorporated. Keep working the mixture until it becomes fluffy and creamy.

4. If dough is too stiff, add the warm milk, a tablespoon at a time, until the mixture is softer.

5. Using a tablespoon or cookie scoop, drop twenty-four balls on a parchment-lined baking sheet.

6. Sprinkle the garnish on the center of each dough ball and flatten to ⅓ inch.

7. Bake until light golden, 15–16 minutes. Transfer to a wire rack to cool.

CHAPTER TWELVE

RECIPES TO HELP CHANGE THE COURSE OF PARKINSON'S DISEASE

A well-balanced diet improves your gut health and increases your ability to prevent or manage Parkinson's. I emphasize lean protein, beans, and legumes, as well as whole grains. Balance those with an assortment of fresh fruits and vegetables—especially glucoraphanin-rich cruciferous vegetables such as cauliflower, cabbage, kale, cress, bok choy, broccoli, and Brussels sprouts, which also help prevent or manage Parkinson's.[1] And enjoy a cup of brewed tea with your meal because higher intake of tea has been associated with a lower risk of Parkinson's disease.[2]

INDIAN LENTIL SOUP

This versatile soup, known as dal, is a staple of Indian cooking. My kids have this dish almost daily. The spices can be adjusted to make it as flavorful or mild as you wish, but remember that the spices in this recipe are anti-inflammatory, and lowering inflammation may be a key to preventing Parkinson's.[3] Dal is great on a wintry day, and with a little extra simmering to reduce the liquid it makes a wonderful sauce over rice or cooked vegetables. Red lentils are low in fat and high in fiber, promoting gut integrity. They are also rich in protein as well as the B vitamins the brain needs to function optimally.

Servings: 4

Ingredients

    1 tablespoon olive oil

    1 small onion, diced

    1 teaspoon cumin seeds

    1 teaspoon ground cumin

    1 teaspoon ground turmeric

    1 teaspoon curry powder

    1 teaspoon garam masala

    1 teaspoon salt

    ½ teaspoon cayenne (or to taste)

    1 large bay leaf (or 2 small)

    1 green chile, diced (optional)

    1 cup red lentils

    4 cups water

    Cilantro (optional)

Instructions

1. Heat oil in a medium saucepan over medium heat. Add onion and cumin seeds and sauté until the onion is translucent.

2. Add the ground cumin, turmeric, curry, garam masala, salt, cayenne, bay leaf, and green chile (if using).

3. Cook for about a minute, stirring often, until spices become aromatic.

4. Add the red lentils and stir well.

5. Add the water. Bring to a boil, then reduce heat and simmer, covered, approximately 30 minutes.

6. Garnish with cilantro and additional green chile, if desired.

CHICKEN AND WATERCRESS WRAP

This wrap is a delicious source of lean protein and a way to up your daily intake of cruciferous vegetables. Avocado and olive oil provide good fats. Studies have shown that "eating peppers twice or more per week was consistently associated with at least 30 percent reduced risk of developing Parkinson's disease."[4] And do not forget the olives! Researchers are finding that a compound in olives, hydroxytyrosol, helps support dopamine levels and may significantly ease Parkinson's motor symptoms.[5]

Servings: 2

Ingredients

1 chicken breast, cut into small chunks

Salt

Black pepper

1 tablespoon olive oil

1 garlic clove, finely chopped

1 small handful grated mozzarella

2 large whole-wheat tortillas

1 red pepper, sliced

1 red onion, finely sliced

½ teaspoon red pepper flakes

15 olives (black or green), pitted and cut into quarters

1 avocado, sliced

1 handful watercress

1 handful spinach

A few basil leaves, torn

Dressing

1 tablespoon honey

1 tablespoon whole-grain mustard

Instructions

1. Season the chicken with salt and pepper.

2. In a frying pan, heat the oil over high heat and fry the chicken until browned on all sides and cooked through, approximately 4 minutes.

3. Reduce the heat to medium and add the garlic. Cook, stirring, until the garlic is softened, but take care not to burn it.

4. Put a thin layer of the grated mozzarella on the tortillas.

5. Spoon the chicken mixture on top of the cheese and top with the red pepper, onion, red pepper flakes, olives, avocado, watercress, spinach, and basil.

6. In a small bowl, whisk together the honey and mustard. Drizzle the dressing over the filling and roll up each tortilla, tucking in the sides like a burrito.

7. Cook the wraps in a dry, medium-hot frying pan for 2–3 minutes each side, using another pan to weigh the wraps down.

DR. NANDI'S NO-COOK PUMPKIN OATMEAL

Oatmeal is high in fiber and a prebiotic food that can be prepared in many ways. I like to combine it with pumpkin butter and warm spices. The chia seeds add a little extra fiber and give the oatmeal a nice texture. And chia seeds absorb up to thirty times their weight in water; this water is released in digestion and can help you maintain hydration. Pepitas (hulled raw pumpkin seeds) are anti-inflammatory, and bananas are an effortless way to add potassium, which helps reduce neuroinflammation.

Servings: 1

Ingredients
¼ cup quick oats
¾ cup unsweetened almond milk
2 tablespoons pumpkin butter (see page 204)
1 teaspoon chia seeds
Cinnamon
Pumpkin pie spice
¼ banana, sliced
1 tablespoon pepitas

Directions
1. Mix the oats and ½ cup of the almond milk in a jar.

PUMPKIN BUTTER

This delicious pumpkin butter adds fiber, vitamins, an anti-inflammatory boost, and a dollop of calcium, potassium, and magnesium to your meals—which I believe are all useful nutrients in preventing Parkinson's. It is great in oatmeal as well as on toast, yogurt, granola, pancakes, graham crackers, and baked sweet potatoes. Stored in an airtight container, it will keep in the refrigerator for two weeks and in the freezer for up to six months.

Makes about 4 cups

Ingredients

- 3½ cups pumpkin puree (canned will work)
- 2 teaspoons vanilla extract
- ¾ cup organic apple cider
- 1 cup (packed) organic brown sugar, or ⅔ cup date sugar
- 3 cinnamon sticks
- 1–2 teaspoons pumpkin pie spice

Directions

1. Mix pumpkin, vanilla, apple cider, sugar, cinnamon sticks, and pumpkin pie spice in a large saucepan.
2. Bring mixture to a boil over high heat.
3. Reduce the heat and simmer, stirring frequently, until thickened, 30–40 minutes.
4. Cool completely and store in an airtight container.

2. Stir in the pumpkin butter, chia seeds, a pinch of cinnamon, and a pinch of pumpkin pie spice.

3. Add banana. Cover the jar, shake, and refrigerate overnight.

4. The next day, remove from the refrigerator and let sit on the counter for 30 minutes to warm up.

5. Stir in the remaining ¼ cup of almond milk, sprinkle with a little more cinnamon and pumpkin pie spice, and top with pepitas.

BEAN SALAD

Beans have been shown to have neuroprotective benefits.[6] If you have the time, soaking and cooking dried beans tends to be not only less expensive but also more nutritious than using canned beans, with more fiber, iron, potassium, protein, and magnesium. Fortunately, canned beans have nearly as many benefits, but when shopping, pay attention to the label and look for low-sodium varieties with fewer preservatives. (If you can't find low-sodium beans, be sure to rinse the beans very well—you will still receive plenty of benefits.)

Servings: 4

Ingredients

¾ cup olive oil

¼ cup red wine vinegar

1¼ tablespoons sugar, or ½ cup finely minced dates

3 cloves garlic, peeled and minced

1¼ teaspoons salt

1¼ teaspoons ground cumin

1¼ teaspoons chili powder

⅓ teaspoon black pepper

4 cups cooked basmati rice

22 ounces cooked kidney beans, rinsed and drained

18 ounces cooked fava beans, rinsed and drained

2 cups corn kernels, fresh or frozen and thawed

6 green onions, thinly sliced

1 medium red pepper, seeded and chopped

⅓ cup minced cilantro

Directions

1. In a large mixing bowl, whisk together the oil, vinegar, sugar, garlic, salt, cumin, chili powder, and pepper.
2. Add the remaining ingredients. Toss to coat evenly.
3. Chill for 1 hour and serve cool.

AFTERWORD

began writing this book soon after my father died. I have struggled with my father's death, and because of that struggle, I am determined to help others in my position, in my father's position, and in my family's position to avoid the tragedy that should have never been. My dad did not deserve for the last decade of his life to turn out like it did. I am happy I had that time with him, but I believe if I had known then what I know now, it could have been far more fulfilling.

Many will say of patients suffering from stroke, Alzheimer's, or Parkinson's disease, "They're old. There's nothing you can do about it." It seems as if once people are deemed to be elderly, they are thought to be discardable, and instead of offering them the goal of healing or hope, many of us utter platitudes like *They've lived a good life. This is what happens. It is a consequence of age.*

I am here to say this is not necessarily the case, because I have seen so many active, thriving eighty-year-olds and some ninety-year-olds. The world is changing, and so is the length of time we can expect to have a good quality of life. But to achieve that, it is imperative that we change our mindset. With a changed mindset comes an understanding that not only can we treat stroke, Alzheimer's, and Parkinson's, but we can also prevent them and give people hope that their lives do not have to be filled with this kind of despair and struggle.

I have found that aging, even after a severe illness, can be better than advertised. The evidence is more exciting than I thought it would be. I was hopeful that to the tools of traditional medicine we could add the Five Pillars, but then I found that the gut microbiome, which can be changed relatively easily, can be a weapon against these diseases. The more information I found about how the gut really affects the brain, the more I saw that we can make specific changes to the gut.

In writing this book, I hope not only to help folks prevent disease for themselves or their loved ones but also to help them after the event, to hopefully offer a better future, limit damage, and even reverse some of the damage that may have already occurred. I find it fulfilling personally and also at a community level because my goal as a doctor has always been to help people achieve a better life in whatever way I can. This book has satisfied that dream in both traditional and nontraditional ways. I am not putting a stethoscope on the reader or performing a procedure, but by imparting knowledge and being able to share tools to make some of these changes to help heal, I am hoping to contribute to your and your family's health.

I can see a future in which, when people present with neurological issues, the gut is the first line of defense and a mainstay of treatment instead of a sidebar. This will be a wonderful day, not just for me personally but for patients and their families as well.

GLOSSARY

BBB Blood-brain barrier. A cellular wall designed to protect the brain from potentially damaging toxins, pathogens, and inflammation circulating in the bloodstream.

Butyrate Butyrate is a naturally occurring fatty acid in your body.

Cortisol The hormone produced by the adrenal glands and regulated by the pituitary gland; regulates stress response.

Dysbiosis Imbalance in the gut.

ENS Enteric nervous system. The lining of the digestive tract has millions of neurons (nerve cells).[1]

GI barrier Gastrointestinal barrier. The mucosal lining of the gut, essential to filtering through the barrage of substances that can enter the gut.

Glycemic index (GI) A scale quantifying the effect of a food on a person's blood sugar levels.

Gut-brain axis The vast and complex neurological and biochemical system bidirectionally connecting the gut and the brain.

Gut microbiome The trillions of bacteria and other microorganisms that naturally live within the intestines to help us digest our food.

Inflammation A normal part of the body's response to an irritant.

Leaky gut   The concept of relative intestinal permeability, or
                           the ability for things to move through the intestinal
                           lining.

Lewy bodies   Lewy bodies are sticky protein clusters that can
                           disrupt brain function.

Metabolites   Substances produced during metabolism, which
                           is the process of breaking down foods, drugs, or
                           chemicals.

Metabolize   Chemical reactions in the body's cells that change
                           food into energy.

Microbiota   The collection of microorganisms living in a defined
                           environment, such as the digestive tract.

Neurodegeneration   Conditions that gradually damage and destroy
                           parts of your nervous system, including the brain.

Postbiotics   The products probiotics secrete as they break down
                           fiber. These help support the immune system,
                           stabilize blood sugar, and alleviate symptoms of
                           irritable bowel syndrome.

Prebiotics   Foods that act as the food for the human
                           microorganisms in the gut.

Probiotics   Probiotics are the beneficial bacteria that naturally
                           occur in your body, particularly in the gut. These
                           live microorganisms help regulate digestion and
                           intestinal function.

SCFA   Short-chain fatty acid.

ACKNOWLEDGMENTS

To my father, Uma Shankar Nandi, my original hero, whose unconditional love gave me the strength I needed throughout my life. His brilliance, dedication, wisdom, and empathy lifted up my family. I dedicate this work to my dad and hope that it helps others avoid the pain that he suffered in his last years of life.

To my beautiful mother, Sikha Nandi, my first love, I owe everything. I lost my dear mother while writing this book. Her unwavering spirit and fierce wisdom inspired and encouraged me throughout my life. She would have loved this book, and I am sure she would have devoured it from cover to cover with fervent interest. Mama, this one is for your Buru!

My wife, Kali, whose inspirational words and unwavering support are instrumental in my life. She encourages, invigorates, and lifts up our family with her beautiful soul. As I wrote this book, she gave me the guidance and space needed to fulfill my dream.

My sister, Mohua, who shared my wonderful father with me. From the day he suffered his stroke, her extraordinary care and dedication to him were inspirational and exceptional. Without her perseverance and advocacy, my father would have suffered far more. She is an angel and I am forever thankful for her.

My children, Partha, Shaan, Rakhi, and Charley. They inspire me each day to be a better father and person and help me to understand the true meaning of love and support. As I worked on this book, they shared their pride and enthusiasm, understanding how important it was to help others not have the same fate as their grandpa.

Alice Peck, thank you for turning this dream into reality. Your brilliance and dedication are rare. With your help, so many will be inspired to prevent and heal their mind, gut, and bodies. Namaste!

To my agent, Michele Martin, thank you for your guidance and leadership. You helped me understand the importance of this deeply personal work. Your advocacy is truly special. I feel privileged to call you my friend.

My editor, Daniela Rapp, thank you for your guidance. Thank you for your empathy and support, understanding the pain of a son whose father and hero is taken away from him.

NOTES

INTRODUCTION

1. M. Hasan Mohajeri et al., "Relationship Between the Gut Microbiome and Brain Function," *Nutrition Reviews* 76, no. 7 (2018): 481–496; John F. Cryan and Timothy G. Dinan, "Mind-Altering Microorganisms: The Impact of the Gut Microbiota on Brain and Behaviour," *Nature Reviews Neuroscience* 13, no. 10 (2012): 701–712.

2. Barbara Caracciolo et al., "Cognitive Decline, Dietary Factors and Gut-Brain Interactions," *Mechanisms of Ageing and Development* 136 (2014): 59–69; Aimée Parker, Sonia Fonseca, and Simon R. Carding, "Gut Microbes and Metabolites as Modulators of Blood-Brain Barrier Integrity and Brain Health," *Gut Microbes* 11, no. 2 (2020): 135–157.

3. R. N. Kalaria, R. Akinyemi, and M. Ihara, "Stroke Injury, Cognitive Impairment and Vascular Dementia," *Biochimica et Biophysica Acta* 1862, no. 5 (2016): 915–925, doi: 10.1016/j.bbadis.2016.01.015.

4. Dag Aarsland and Martin Wilhelm Kurz, "The Epidemiology of Dementia Associated with Parkinson Disease," *Journal of the Neurological Sciences* 289, no. 1–2 (2010): 18–22, https://www.science direct.com/science/article/abs/pii/S0022510X09008193.

5. Hui Wang et al., "Genetic and Environmental Factors in Alzheimer's and Parkinson's Diseases and Promising Therapeutic Intervention via Fecal Microbiota Transplantation," *NPJ Parkinson's Disease* 7, no. 1 (2021): 70; Gad Abraham, Loes Rutten-Jacobs, and Michael Inouye, "Risk Prediction Using Polygenic Risk Scores for Prevention of Stroke and Other Cardiovascular Diseases," *Stroke* 52, no. 9 (2021): 2983–2991; Kevin Roe, "An Alternative Explanation for Alzheimer's Disease and Parkinson's Disease Initiation from Specific Antibiotics, Gut Microbiota Dysbiosis and Neurotoxins," *Neurochemical Research* 47, no. 3 (2022): 517–530; Judy Potashkin et al., "Understanding the Links Between Cardiovascular Disease and Parkinson's Disease," *Movement Disorders* 35, no. 1 (2020): 55–74; Abolfazl Avan and Vladimir Hachinski, "Stroke and Dementia, Leading Causes of Neurological Disability and Death, Potential for Prevention," *Alzheimer's and Dementia* 17, no. 6 (2021): 1072–1076.

6. P. Turnbaugh et al., "The Human Microbiome Project," *Nature* 449 (2007): 804–810, https://doi.org/10.1038/nature06244.

7. Yaohua Chen et al., "Defining Brain Health: A Concept Analysis," *International Journal of Geriatric Psychiatry* 37, no. 1 (2022); Tanya T. Nguyen et al., "Association of Loneliness and Wisdom with Gut Microbial Diversity and Composition: An Exploratory Study," *Frontiers in Psychiatry* 12 (2021): 395; Michelle Guan et al., "Improved Psychosocial Measures Associated with Physical Activity May Be Explained by Alterations in Brain-Gut Microbiome Signatures," *Scientific Reports* 13, no. 1 (2023): 10332.

8. P. A. Boyle et al., "Effect of a Purpose in Life on Risk of Incident Alzheimer Disease and Mild Cognitive Impairment in Community-Dwelling Older Persons," *Archives of General Psychiatry* 67, no. 3 (2010): 304–310.

9. Roma Bhatia et al., "Social Networks, Social Support, and Life Expectancy in Older Adults: the Cardiovascular Health Study," *Archives of Gerontology and Geriatrics* 111 (2023): 104981, https://doi.org/10.1016/j.archger.2023.104981.

10. Sarah D. Pressman, Tara Kraft, and Stephanie Bowlin, "Well-Being: Physical, Psychological, and Social," in *Encyclopedia of Behavioral Medicine,* eds. Marc D. Gellman and J. Rick Turner (New York: Springer International Publishing, 2020), 2334–2339; Gholam Rasul Mohammad Rahimi et al., "Effects of Lifestyle Intervention on Inflammatory Markers and Waist Circumference in Overweight/Obese Adults with Metabolic Syndrome: A Systematic Review and Meta-analysis of Randomized Controlled Trials," *Biological Research for Nursing* 24, no. 1 (2022): 94–105; L. Greene-Higgs et al., "Social Network Diversity and the Daily Burden of Inflammatory Bowel Disease," *Clinical and Translational Gastroenterology* 14, no. 5 (2023): e00572, https://pubmed.ncbi.nlm.nih.gov/36854057/#:~:text=Results:%20Patients%20with%20IBD%20with,a%20low%20degree%20of%20loneliness.

11. Herbert Benson, *Beyond the Relaxation Response: The Stress-Reduction Program That Has Helped Millions of Americans* (New York: Harmony/Rodale, 2019).

12. Y. Sun et al., "Alteration of Faecal Microbiota Balance Related to Long-Term Deep Meditation," *General Psychiatry* 36, no. 1 (2023): e100893, doi: 10.1136/gpsych-2022-100893.

13. Patricia L. Gerbarg et al., "The Effect of Breathing, Movement, and Meditation on Psychological and Physical Symptoms and Inflammatory Biomarkers in Inflammatory Bowel Disease: A Randomized Controlled Trial," *Inflammatory Bowel Diseases* 21, no. 12 (2015): 2886–2896; Sun et al., "Alteration of Faecal Microbiota," e100893.

14. Z. Xie et al., "Healthy Human Fecal Microbiota Transplantation into Mice Attenuates MPTP-Induced Neurotoxicity via AMPK/SOD2 Pathway," *Aging and Disease* 14, no. 6 (December 1, 2023): 2193–2214, doi: 10.14336/AD.2023.0309/; Judith Metzdorf and Lars Tönges, "Short-Chain Fatty Acids in the Context of Parkinson's Disease," *Neural Regeneration Research* 16, no. 10 (2021): 2015–2016, https:// www.ncbi.nlm.nih.gov/pmc/articles/PMC8343296/.

15. National Institutes of Health, US Department of Health and Human Services, *Opportunities and Challenges in Digestive Diseases Research: Recommendations of the National Commission on Digestive Diseases,* NIH Publication 08-6514 (Bethesda, MD: National Institutes of Health, 2009).

CHAPTER 1: WHAT HAPPENS IN THE GUT DOES NOT NECESSARILY STAY IN THE GUT

1. P. Turnbaugh et al., "An Obesity-Associated Gut Microbiome with Increased Capacity for Energy Harvest," *Nature* 444 (2006): 1027–1031, https://doi.org/10.1038/nature05414.

2. Turnbaugh et al., "An Obesity-Associated Gut Microbiome with Increased Capacity for Energy Harvest," 2006.

3. Zahra Bayrami et al., "Functional Foods and Dietary Patterns for Prevention of Cognitive Decline in Aging," in *Nutrients and Nutraceuticals for Active & and Healthy Ageing,* eds. S. M. Nabavi, G. D'Onofrio, and S. F. Nabavi (Singapore: Springer, 2020): 217–238; Nikolaj Travica et al., "The Effect of Blueberry Interventions on Cognitive Performance and Mood: A Systematic Review of Randomized Controlled Trials," *Brain, Behavior, and Immunity* 85 (2020): 96–105.

4. University of Exeter, "Blueberry Concentrate Improves Brain Function in Older People," *Science Daily,* March 7, 2017, www.sciencedaily.com /releases/2017/03/170307100356.

5. C. W. Zhu et al., "Five Blueberry Anthocyanins and Their Antioxidant, Hypoglycemic, and Hypolipidemic Effects *in Vitro,*" *Frontiers in Nutrition* 10 (2023): 1172982, doi: 10.3389/fnut.2023.1172982.

6. J. Tan et al., "The Role of Short-Chain Fatty Acids in Health and Disease," *Advances in Immunology* 121 (2014): 91–119, doi: 10.1016/ B978-0-12-800100-4.00003-9.

7. Michael J. Federle and Bonnie L. Bassler, "Interspecies Communication in Bacteria," *Journal of Clinical Investigation* 112, no. 9 (2003): 1291–1299, https://www.ncbi.nlm.nih.gov/pmc/articles/PMC228483/.

8. M. I. McBurney, "The Gut: Central Organ in Nutrient Requirements and Metabolism," *Canadian Journal of Physiology and Pharmacology* 72, no. 3 (1994): 260–265, https://pubmed.ncbi.nlm.nih.gov/8069772 /#:~:text=The%20gut%20is%20an%20important,any%20tissue%20 in%20the%20body.

9. Sigrid Breit et al., "Vagus Nerve as Modulator of the Brain–Gut Axis in Psychiatric and Inflammatory Disorders," *Frontiers in Psychiatry* 9, no. 44 (2018), https://www.ncbi.nlm.nih.gov/pmc/articles/PMC585 9128/#:~:text=The%20vagus%20nerve%20is%20responsible,%2C%20 and%20vomiting%20(17).

10. "What Defines a Neurotransmitter?" in D. Purves et al., eds., *Neuroscience*, 2nd ed. (Sunderland, MA: Sinauer Associates, 2001), https://www.ncbi.nlm.nih.gov/books/NBK10957/#:~:text=As%20 briefly%20described%20in%20the,terminals%20into%20the%20 synaptic%20cleft; Natalie Terry and Kara Gross Margolis, "Serotonergic Mechanisms Regulating the GI Tract: Experimental Evidence and Therapeutic Relevance," in *Gastrointestinal Pharmacology*, vol. 239 of *Handbook of Experimental Pharmacology*, ed. Beverley Greenwood-Van Meerveld (Springer International Publishing, 2017), 319–342, https://www.ncbi.nlm.nih.gov/pmc/articles /PMC5526216/#:~:text=Serotonin%20(5%2Dhydroxytryptamine %3B%205,%2C%20paracrine%2C%20and%20endocrine%20 actions.

11. Bashar W. Badran et al., "Neurophysiologic Effects of Transcutaneous Auricular Vagus Nerve Stimulation (taVNS) via Electrical Stimulation of the Tragus: A Concurrent taVNS/fMRI Study and Review," *Brain Stimulation* 11, no. 3 (2018): 492–500.

12. Sophie J. Müller et al., "Vagus Nerve Stimulation Increases Stomach-Brain Coupling via a Vagal Afferent Pathway," *Brain Stimulation* 15, no. 5 (2022): 1279–1289; "5 Ways to Stimulate Your Vagus Nerve," *Cleveland Clinic*, March 10, 2022, https://health.clevelandclinic.org /vagus-nerve-stimulation.

13. Juliana Durack and Susan V. Lynch, "The Gut Microbiome: Relationships with Disease and Opportunities for Therapy," *Journal of Experimental Medicine* 216, no.1 (2019): 20–40, https://www.ncbi.nlm .nih.gov/pmc/articles/PMC6314516/.

14. Ewen Callaway, "C-Section Babies Are Missing Key Microbes," *Nature,* September 18, 2019, doi: 10.1038/d41586-019-02807-x.

15. E. K. Mallott et al., "Human Microbiome Variation Associated with Race and Ethnicity Emerges as Early as 3 Months of Age," *PLoS Biology* 21, no. 8 (2023): e3002230, https://doi.org/10.1371/journal .pbio.3002230.

16. Shaohui Geng et al., "Gut Microbiota Are Associated with Psychological Stress-Induced Defections in Intestinal and Blood-Brain Barriers," *Frontiers in Microbiology* 10 (2020): 3067.

CHAPTER 2: GUT HEALTH: A STATE OF DIS-EASE

1. "Gut Troubles: Pain, Gassiness, Bloating, and More," *NIH News in Health,* February 2020, https://newsinhealth.nih.gov/2020/02/gut

troubles#:~:text=Around%2060%20to%2070%20million,treat%20
when%20they%20first%20develop.

2. Jotham Suez et al., "Personalized Microbiome-Driven Effects of Non-Nutritive Sweeteners on Human Glucose Tolerance," *Cell* 185, no. 18 (2022): 3307–3328.

3. "Polyunsaturated Fats," *American Heart Association,* last reviewed October 25, 2023, https://www.heart.org/en/healthy-living/healthy-eating/eat-smart/fats/polyunsaturated-fats.

4. "Dietary Fat: Know Which to Choose," *Mayo Clinic,* February 15, 2023, https://www.mayoclinic.org/healthy-lifestyle/nutrition-and-healthy-eating/in-depth/fat/art-20045550.

5. Nathalie T. Bendsen et al., "Effect of Industrially Produced Trans Fat on Markers of Systemic Inflammation: Evidence from a Randomized Trial in Women," *Journal of Lipid Research* 52, no. 10 (2011): 1821–1828, https://www.sciencedirect.com/science/article/pii/S0022227520408466#:~:text=In%20cross%2Dsectional%20studies%2C%20intake,1%2C%202%2C%203).

6. A. Dona and I. S. Arvanitoyannis, "Health Risks of Genetically Modified Foods," *Critical Reviews in Food Science and Nutrition* 49, no. 2 (2009): 164–175, doi: 10.1080/10408390701855993; A. Bakhsh et al., "Genetically Modified Organisms in Europe: State of Affairs, Birth, Research, and the Regulatory Process(es)," in *Genetically Modified Organisms in Food Production: Risk and Benefits,* ed. Abdur Rashid, (New York: Academic Press, 2023), 165–172.

7. P. Nandi, "Toxic Ingredients to Avoid," *Ask Dr. Nandi,* July 16, 2018, https://askdrnandi.com/toxic-ingredients-to-avoid/.

8. D. Partridge et al., "Food Additives: Assessing the Impact of Exposure to Permitted Emulsifiers on Bowel and Metabolic Health—Introducing the FADiets Study," *Nutrition Bulletin* 44, no. 4 (2019): 329–349, https://doi.org/10.1111/nbu.12408.

9. Leonie Elizabeth et al., "Ultra-Processed Foods and Health Outcomes: A Narrative Review," *Nutrients* 12, no. 7 (2020): 1955.

10. A. E. Bender, "Nutritional Aspects of Frozen Foods," *Agricultural and Food Sciences* (1993): 123–140, doi: 10.1007/978-1-4615-3550-8_5.

11. C. M. Benbrook and D. R. Davis, "The Dietary Risk Index System: A Tool to Track Pesticide Dietary Risks," *Environmental Health* 19 (2020): 103, https://doi.org/10.1186/s12940-020-00657-z.

12. Benbrook and Davis, "The Dietary Risk Index System," 103.

13. Elizabeth et al., "Ultra-Processed Foods," 1955.

14. Mark Lown, "Prolonged Antibiotic Use, Inflammation and Obesity (PROBITY)—A Retrospective Cohort Study," *NIHR School for Primary Care Research,* n.d. (accessed November 28, 2023), https://www.spcr.nihr.ac.uk/research/projects/prolonged-antibiotic-use-inflammation-and-obesity-probity-a-retrospective-cohort-study.

15. Tera L. Fazzino, "The Reinforcing Natures of Hyper-Palatable Foods: Behavioral Evidence for Their Reinforcing Properties and the Role of the US Food Industry in Promoting Their Availability," *Current Addiction Reports* 9, no. 4 (2022): 298–306.

16. University of Copenhagen, Faculty of Health and Medical Sciences, "The Composition of Gut Bacteria Almost Recovers After Antibiotics," *Science Daily*, October 23, 2018, www.sciencedaily.com/releases/2018/10/181023110545.htm.

17. Vincenzo Monda et al., "Exercise Modifies the Gut Microbiota with Positive Health Effects," *Oxidative Medicine and Cellular Longevity* 2017 (2017): 3831972, https://www.ncbi.nlm.nih.gov/pmc/articles/PMC5357536/#:~:text=Exercise%20is%20able%20to%20enrich,mucosal%20immunity%20and%20improve%20barrier.

18. Ron Grossman and Charles Leroux, "A New 'Roseto Effect': 'People Are Nourished by Other People,'" *Chicago Tribune*, October 11, 1996.

19. Beckman Institute, "Keep Your Friends Close, Cortisol Levels Low for Life," *Science Daily*, June 30, 2021, https://www.sciencedaily.com/releases/2021/06/210630173629.htm.

20. Annelise Madison and Janice K. Kiecolt-Glaser, "Stress, Depression, Diet, and the Gut Microbiota: Human-Bacteria Interactions at the Core of Psychoneuroimmunology and Nutrition," *Current Opinion in Behavioral Sciences* 28, no. 3 (2019): 105–110, https://doi.org/10.1016/j.cobeha.2019.01.011.

21. Sir William Osler, "Books and Men," *Boston Medical and Surgical Journal* 144 (1901): 60-61.

CHAPTER 3: HOW TO CHANGE YOUR GUT HEALTH

1. Emanuele Rinninella et al., "Food Components and Dietary Habits: Keys for a Healthy Gut Microbiota Composition," *Nutrients* 11, no. 10 (2019): 2393.

2. Jie Gao, Faizan Ahmed Sadiq, Yixin Zheng, et al., "Biofilm-Based Delivery Approaches and Specific Enrichment Strategies of Probiotics in the Human Gut," *Gut Microbes* 14, no. 1 (2022): 2126274, doi: 10.1080/19490976.2022.2126274.

3. Loris Riccardo Lopetuso et al., "The Therapeutic Management of Gut Barrier Leaking: The Emerging Role for Mucosal Barrier Protectors," *European Review for Medical and Pharmacological Sciences* 9, no. 6 (2015): 1068–1076.

4. Ning Zhang, Xuesong Huang, Yanhua Zeng, et al., "Study on Prebiotic Effectiveness of Neutral Garlic Fructan in Vitro," *Food Science and Human Wellness* 2, no. 3–4 (2013): 119–123.

5. R. Slimestad, T. Fossen, and I. M. Vågen, "Onions: A Source of Unique Dietary Flavonoids," *Journal of Agricultural and Food Chemistry* 55, no. 25 (2007): 10067–10080, doi: 10.1021/jf0712503.

6. Y. Shukla and M. Singh, "Cancer Preventative Properties of Ginger: A Brief Review," *Food and Chemical Toxicology* 45, no. 5 (May 2007): 683–690, https://doi.org/10.1016/j.fct.2006.11.002.

7. Fiona Frederike Cox et al., "Protective Effects of Curcumin in Cardiovascular Diseases—Impact on Oxidative Stress and Mitochondria," *Cells* 11, no. 3 (2022): 342, https://www.ncbi.nlm.nih.gov/pmc/articles/PMC8833931/; Gary W. Small et al., "Memory and Brain Amyloid and Tau Effects of a Bioavailable Form of Curcumin in Non-Demented Adults: A Double-Blind, Placebo-Controlled 18-Month Trial," *The American Journal of Geriatric Psychiatry* 26, no. 3 (2018): 266–277, https://www.sciencedirect.com/science/article/pii/S1064748117305110?via%3Dihub.

8. Susan J. Hewlings and Douglas S. Kalman, "Curcumin: A Review of Its Effects on Human Health," *Foods* 6, no. 10 (2017): 92, https://www.ncbi.nlm.nih.gov/pmc/articles/PMC5664031/#:~:text=There%20are%20several%20components%20that,agents%20provides%20multiple%20health%20benefits.

9. Harvard T.H. Chan School of Public Health, "Yogurt," The Nutrition Source, https://www.hsph.harvard.edu/nutritionsource/food-features/yogurt/#:~:text=Yogurt%20and%20Health,-Yogurt%20offers%20several&text=%5B%5D%20It%20has%20been%20proposed,ulcerative%20colitis%2C%20and%20rheumatoid%20arthritis.

10. Navindra P. Seeram, "Berry Fruits: Compositional Elements, Biochemical Activities, and the Impact of Their Intake on Human Health, Performance, and Disease," *Journal of Agricultural and Food Chemistry* 56, no. 3 (2008): 627–629, https://doi.org/10.1021/jf071988k.

11. V. Monda et al., "Exercise Modifies the Gut Microbiota with Positive Health Effects," *Oxidative Medicine and Cellular Longevity* (2017), doi: 10.1155/2017/3831972.

12. Jacob M. Allen et al., "Exercise Alters Gut Microbiota Composition and Function in Lean and Obese Humans," *Medicine and Science in Sports Exercise* 50, no. 4 (2018): 747–757.

13. Mandy Oaklander, "The Happy Effect Exercise Has on . . . Your Gut Bacteria?," *Prevention*, June 9, 2014, https://www.prevention.com/life/a20473561/exercise-makes-your-gut-bacteria-more-diverse/.

14. L. Strate et al., "Physical Activity Decreases Diverticular Complications," *American Journal of Gastroenterology* 104, no. 5 (May 2009): 1221-1230, doi: 10.1038/ajg.2009.121; "Exercise Shown to Release Protein, Reducing Bowel Cancer Risk," Newcastle University Press Office, April 7, 2022, https://www.ncl.ac.uk/press/articles/archive/2022/04/exercisereducesbowelcancerrisk/#:~:text=Bowel%20cancer%20prevalence%20It%20is%20estimated%20that,tasks%20or%20work%20like%20gardening%20or%20cleaning.

15. Siobhan F. Clarke et al., "Exercise and Associated Dietary Extremes Impact on Gut Microbial Diversity," *Gut* 63, no. 12 (2014): 1913–1920.
16. Tanja Sobko et al., "Impact of Outdoor Nature-Related Activities on Gut Microbiota, Fecal Serotonin, and Perceived Stress in Preschool Children: The Play & Grow Randomized Controlled Trial," *Scientific Reports* 10, no. 1 (2020): 21993.
17. Ayman Zaky Elsamanoudy et al., "The Role of Nutrition Related Genes and Nutrigenetics in Understanding the Pathogenesis of Cancer," *Journal of Microscopy and Ultrastructure* 4, no. 3 (2016): 115–122, doi: 10.1016/j.jmau.2016.02.002.
18. Elsamanoudy et al., "The Role of Nutrition," 2016.
19. Ravinder Nagpal et al., "Gut Microbiome and Aging: Physiological and Mechanistic Insights," *Nutrition and Healthy Aging* 4, no. 4 (2018): 267–285, doi: 10.3233/NHA-170030.
20. Agata Białecka-Dębek et al., "Gut Microbiota, Probiotic Interventions, and Cognitive Function in the Elderly: A Review of Current Knowledge," *Nutrients* 13, no. 8 (2021): 2514.

CHAPTER 4: HOW GUT HEALTH CONTRIBUTES TO STROKE

1. Angela Oldenburg, "Stroke—Symptoms and Causes," *Mayo Clinic,* May 3, 2021, https://www.mayoclinichealthsystem.org/hometown -health/speaking-of-health/stroke-what-it-is-and-the-different-types; Konrad C. Nau et al., "Is It Stroke, or Something Else?," *Journal of Family Practice* 59, no. 1 (January 2010): 26–30.
2. "Stroke Facts," *CDC,* last reviewed May 4, 2023, https://www.cdc.gov /stroke/facts.htm#:~:text=High%20blood%20pressure%2C%20high %20cholesterol,are%20leading%20causes%20of%20stroke; "Stroke: Causes and Risk Factors," *NIH,* last updated May 26, 2023, https:// www.nhlbi.nih.gov/health/stroke/causes; "Know Your Risk for Stroke," *CDC,* last reviewed May 4, 2023, https://www.cdc.gov/stroke/risk _factors.htm.
3. N. Li et al., "Change of Intestinal Microbiota in Cerebral Ischemic Stroke Patients," *BMC Microbiology* 19 (2019): 191, https://doi.org/10 .1186/s12866-019-1552-1.
4. Shengnan Han et al., "A Study of the Correlation between Stroke and Gut Microbiota Over the Last 20 Years: A Bibliometric Analysis," *Frontiers in Microbiology* 14 (2023): 1191758.
5. "Transient Ischemic Attack (TIA)," *Mayo Clinic,* March 26, 2022, https://www.mayoclinic.org/diseases-conditions/transient-ischemic -attack/symptoms-causes/syc-20355679.
6. F. F. Ferri, "Metabolic Syndrome," in *Ferri's Clinical Advisor 2021* (Philadelphia: Elsevier, 2021).

7. M. Foroughi et al., "Stroke and Nutrition: A Review of Studies," *International Journal of Preventive Medicine*, Suppl. 2 (May 4, 2013): S165–S179.

8. J. David Spence, "Nutrition and Risk of Stroke," *Nutrients* 11, no. 3 (2019): 647, https://doi.org/10.3390/nu11030647.

9. Zhou-Qing Kang, Ying Yang, and Bo Xiao, "Dietary Saturated Fat Intake and Risk of Stroke: Systematic Review and Dose-Response Meta-Analysis of Prospective Cohort Studies," *Nutrition, Metabolism and Cardiovascular Diseases* 30, no. 2 (February 10, 2020): 179–189, https://doi.org/10.1016/j.numecd.2019.09.028.

10. Marko Novakovic et al., "Role of Gut Microbiota in Cardiovascular Diseases," *World Journal of Cardiology* 12, no. 4 (2020): 110–122, doi: 10.4330/wjc.v12.i4.110.

11. F. P. Cappuccio, "Cardiovascular and Other Effects of Salt Consumption," *Kidney International Supplements* 3, no. 4 (2013): 312–315, doi: 10.1038/kisup.2013.65.

12. Ye Seul Seo et al., "Dietary Carbohydrate Constituents Related to Gut Dysbiosis and Health," *Microorganisms* 8, no. 3 (2020): 427, doi: 10.3390/microorganisms8030427.

13. "The Dangers of Sleep Deprivation," *American Heart Association*, June 2, 2022, www.heart.org/en/news/2020/06/05/the-dangers-of-sleep-deprivation.

14. Marc Fadel et al., "Association between Reported Long Working Hours and History of Stroke in the CONSTANCES Cohort," *Stroke* 50, no. 7 (2019): 1879–1882.

15. Corrie Pelc, "Gut Microbe Strains Linked to More Severe Strokes and Poorer Post-Stroke Recovery," *Medical News Today*, May 4, 2022, www.medicalnewstoday.com/articles/gut-microbe-strains-linked-to-more-severe-strokes-and-poorer-post-stroke-recovery#What-is-a-stroke?

16. Rida Abid Hasan, Andrew Y. Koh, and Ayesha Zia, "The Gut Microbiome and Thromboembolism," *Thrombosis Research* 189 (May 2020): 77–87, doi: 10.1016/j.thromres.2020.03.003.

17. "WVU Researchers Explore Stroke's Effects on Microbiome," *WVU Today*, West Virginia University, March 12, 2019.

18. Katarzyna Z. Kuter et al., "Increased Beta-Hydroxybutyrate Level Is Not Sufficient for the Neuroprotective Effect of Long-Term Ketogenic Diet in an Animal Model of Early Parkinson's Disease. Exploration of Brain and Liver Energy Metabolism Markers," *International Journal of Molecular Sciences* 22, no. 14 (2021): 7556.

19. P. Petakh, V. Oksenych, and A. Kamyshnyi, "The F/B Ratio as a Biomarker for Inflammation in COVID-19 and T2D: Impact of Metformin," *Biomedicine and Pharmacotherapy* 163 (2023): 114892, doi: 10.1016/j.biopha.2023.114892.

20. F. Magne et al., "The Firmicutes/Bacteroidetes Ratio: A Relevant Marker of Gut Dysbiosis in Obese Patients?," *Nutrients* 12, no. 5 (2020): 1474, doi: 10.3390/nu12051474.
21. "WVU Researchers Explore," *WVU Today,* 2019.
22. "WVU Researchers Explore," *WVU Today,* 2019.
23. S. Y. Park et al., "Gut Dysbiosis: A New Avenue for Stroke Prevention and Therapeutics," *Biomedicines* 11, no. 9 (2023): 2352, doi: 10.3390/biomedicines11092352.
24. "WVU Researchers Explore," *WVU Today,* 2019.

CHAPTER 5: CHANGING THE COURSE OF STROKE
1. A. Oniszczuk et al., "Role of Gut Microbiota, Probiotics and Prebiotics in the Cardiovascular Diseases," *Molecules* 26, no. 4 (2021): 1172, doi: 10.3390/molecules26041172.
2. Diana Kwon, "Targeting Gut Microbes May Help Stroke Recovery," *Scientific American,* December 16, 2019, https://www.scientificamerican.com/article/targeting-gut-microbes-may-help-stroke-recovery/.
3. "WVU Researchers Explore Stroke's Effects on Microbiome," *WVU Today,* West Virginia University, March 12, 2019, https://wvutoday.wvu.edu/stories/2019/03/12/wvu-researchers-explore-stroke-s-effects-on-microbiome.
4. "WVU Researchers Explore," *WVU Today,* 2019; A. K. Arya and B. Hu, "Brain-Gut Axis After Stroke," *Brain Circulation* 4, no. 4 (2018): 165–173, doi: 10.4103/bc.bc_32_18; M. Foroughi et al., "Stroke and Nutrition: A Review of Studies," *International Journal of Preventive Medicine,* Suppl. 2 (May 4, 2013): S165–S179.
5. J. Zhao et al., "The Impact of Gut Microbiota on Post-Stroke Management," *Frontiers in Cellular and Infection Microbiology* 11, https://www.ncbi.nlm.nih.gov/pmc/articles/PMC8546011/.
6. J. Zhao et al., "The Impact of Gut Microbiota on Post-Stroke Management."
7. Shuxia Zhang et al., "New Insight into Gut Microbiota and Their Metabolites in Ischemic Stroke: A Promising Therapeutic Target," *Biomedicine and Pharmacotherapy* 162 (2023): 114559, https://doi.org/10.1016/j.biopha.2023.114559.
8. E. Porras-García et al., "Potential Neuroprotective Effects of Fermented Foods and Beverages in Old Age: A Systematic Review," *Frontiers in Nutrition* 10 (2023): 1170841, doi: 10.3389/fnut.2023.1170841.
9. Rebecca Sadler et al., "Short-Chain Fatty Acids Improve Poststroke Recovery via Immunological Mechanisms," *Journal of Neuroscience* 40, no. 5 (2020): 1162–1173.
10. "Will a Banana a Day Keep a Stroke Away? Low Potassium Intake May Increase Stroke Risk," *Science Daily,* American Academy of

Neurology, August 13, 2002, www.sciencedaily.com/releases/2002
/08/020813072509.htm.

11. R. Swaninathan, "Magnesium Metabolism and its Disorders," *The
Clinical Biochemist Reviews* 24, 2 (2003): 47–66, https://www.ncbi.nlm
.nih.gov/pmc/articles/PMC1855626/#:~:text=Magnesium%20
deficiency%20can%20cause%20a,coronary%20heart%20disease%2C
%20and%20osteoporosis.

12. B. Zhao et al., "The Effect of Magnesium Intake on Stroke Incidence:
A Systematic Review and Meta-Analysis with Trial Sequential
Analysis," *Frontiers in Neurology* 10 (2019): 852. doi: 10.3389/fneur
.2019.00852.

13. Hiroyuki Hoshiko et al., "Identification of Leaky Gut-Related Markers
as Indicators of Metabolic Health in Dutch Adults: The Nutrition
Questionnaires Plus (NQplus) Study," *PLoS One* 16, 6 (2021):
e0252936, doi: 10.1371/journal.pone.0252936.

14. V. Sobhani et al., "Islamic Praying Changes Stress-Related Hormones
and Genes," *Journal of Medicine and Life* 15, no. 4 (2022): 483–488, doi:
10.25122/jml-2021-0167; M. Thakur et al., "Impact of Heartfulness
Meditation Practice on Anxiety, Perceived Stress, Well-being, and
Telomere Length," *Frontiers in Psychology* 14 (2023): 1158760, doi:
10.3389/fpsyg.2023.1158760; Peter Fenwick and Andrew Newberg,
"Meditation, Prayer and Healing: A Neuroscience Perspective," in
Spirituality and Psychiatry, 2nd ed., eds. Christopher C. H. Cook and
Andrew Powell (Cambridge: Cambridge University Press, 2022), 207–
219; P. Forte et al., "Mindfulness-Based Stress Reduction in Cancer
Patients: Impact on Overall Survival, Quality of Life and Risk Factor,"
European Review for Medical and Pharmacological Sciences 27, no. 17
(2023).

15. W. Jiang et al., "Alteration of Gut Microbiome and Correlated Lipid
Metabolism in Post-Stroke Depression," *Frontiers in Cellular and
Infection Microbiology* 11 (2021): 663967, doi: 10.3389/fcimb.2021
.663967.

16. Moeka Kamiya, "Rumination and the Gut Microbiome: Effects of a
Brief Mindfulness Intervention," Lawrence University, June 14, 2022,
https://lux.lawrence.edu/cgi/viewcontent.cgi?article=1177&context
=luhp.

17. "How to Practice Mindfulness-Based Stress Reduction (MBSR),"
Calm, December 7, 2024, https://www.calm.com/blog/mindfulness
-based-stress-reduction.

CHAPTER 6: HOW GUT HEALTH CONTRIBUTES TO ALZHEIMER'S DISEASE

1. J. Tokarek et al., "What Is the Role of Gut Microbiota in Obesity
Prevalence? A Few Words about Gut Microbiota and Its Association

with Obesity and Related Diseases," *Microorganisms* 10, no. 1 (December 27; 2021): 52, doi: 10.3390/microorganisms10010052; "Changes in Human Microbiome Precede Alzheimer's Cognitive Decline," National Institute on Aging (July 26, 2023), https://www .nia.nih.gov/news/changes-human-microbiome-precede-alzheimers -cognitive-declines#:~:text=And%2C%20as%20it%20turned%20 out,of%20the%20bacterial%20species%20present; Veronica Lazar et al., "Gut Microbiota, Host Organism, and Diet Trialogue in Diabetes and Obesity," *Frontiers in Nutrition* 6 (2019): 2296–2861, https://www .frontiersin.org/articles/10.3389/fnut.2019.00021/full#:~:text=The%20 disruption%20of%20normal%20microbiota,coordination%20of%20 choline%20availability%2C%20affecting.

2. "Caregiving for a Person with Alzheimer's Disease or a Related Dementia," *CDC,* last reviewed June 30, 2023, https://www.cdc.gov /aging/caregiving/alzheimer.htm#:~:text=The%20majority%20(80%) %20of%20people%20with%20Alzheimer's,year%2C%20more%20 than%2016%20million%20Americans%20provide.

3. "Alzheimer's Disease Fact Sheet," *National Institute on Aging,* April 5, 2023, https://www.nia.nih.gov/health/alzheimers-disease-fact-sheet.

4. "What Happens to the Brain in Alzheimer's Disease?," National Institute on Aging, accessed March 14, 2024, https://www.nia.nih.gov /health/alzheimers-causes-and-risk-factors/what-happens-brain -alzheimers-disease.

5. L. Meda, P. Baron, and G. Scarlato, "Glial Activation in Alzheimer's Disease: The Role of Abeta and Its Associated Proteins," *Neurobiology of Aging* 22, no. 6 (2001): 885–893, doi: 10.1016/s0197-4580(01)00 307-4.

6. "New Culprit in Amyloid Beta Accumulation and Neurodegeneration," Weill Cornell Medicine (November 7, 2023), https://news.weill.cornell .edu/news/2023/11/new-culprit-in-amyloid-beta-accumulation-and -neurodegeneration#:~:text=Researchers%20at%20Weill%20Cornell %20Medicine,vessels%20and%20leads%20to%20neurodegeneration; J. W. Kenney et al., "Inflammation as a Central Mechanism in Alzheimer's Disease," *Alzheimer's and Dementia* 4 (September 6, 2018): 575-590, doi: 10.1016/j.trci.2018.06.014.

7. "How Is Alzheimer's Disease Treated?," National Institute on Aging, September 12, 2023, https://www.nia.nih.gov/health/alzheimers -treatment/how-alzheimers-disease-treated#.

8. "Fiscal Year 2021 Alzheimer's Research Funding," Alzheimer's Impact Movement and Alzheimer's Association, March 2020, https://act.alz .org/site/DocServer/2015_Appropriations_Fact_Sheet__FY16_.pdf ?docID=3641.

9. M. R. Gailani et al., "Relationship between Sunlight Exposure and a Key Genetic Alteration in Basal Cell Carcinoma," *Journal of the National Cancer Institute* 88, no. 6 (1996): 349–354, doi: 10.1093/jnci

/88.6.349; Alekzandrov et al., "Mutational Signatures Associated with Tobacco Smoking in Human Cancer," *Science* 354, no. 6312 (2016): 616–622, doi: 10.1126/science.aag0299.

10. Gabrielle Strobel, "What Is Early Onset Familial Alzheimer Disease (eFAD)?," Alzforum, accessed March 14, 2024, https://www.alzforum .org/early-onset-familial-ad/overview/what-early-onset-familial -alzheimer-disease-efad#:~:text=Definition%3A%20What%20Is%20 eFAD%3F,rarely%20in%20the%20late%20twenties).

11. "What Causes Alzheimer's Disease?," National Institute on Aging, December 24, 2019, https://www.nia.nih.gov/health/alzheimers -causes-and-risk-factors/what-causes-alzheimers-disease#:~:text =The%20number%20of%20people%20with,to%20contribute%20 to%20Alzheimer's%20damage.

12. Nathan H. Johnson et al., "Inflammasome Activation in Traumatic Brain Injury and Alzheimer's Disease," *Translational Research* 254 (2023): 1–12; Z. Guo, L. A. Cupples, A. Kurz et al., "Head Injury and the Risk of ADD in the MIRAGE Study," *Neurology* 54 (March 28, 2000): 1316–23. doi: 10.1212/wnl.54.6.1316.

13. D. J. Berlau et al., "APOE Epsilon2 Is Associated with Intact Cognition but Increased Alzheimer Pathology in the Oldest Old," *Neurology* 72, no. 9 (2009): 829–834, doi: 10.1212/01.wnl.0000343853 .00346.a4.

14. Anum Saeed et al., "Cardiovascular Disease and Alzheimer's Disease: The Heart–Brain Axis," *Journal of the American Heart Association* 12, no. 21 (2023): e030780.

15. "What Is Alzheimer's Disease?," Alzheimer's Association, accessed March 14, 2023, https://www.alz.org/alzheimers-dementia/what-is -alzheimers/causes-and-risk-factors.

16. Mahdieh Golzari-Sorkheh, Donald F. Weaver, and Mark A. Reed, "COVID-19 as a Risk Factor for Alzheimer's Disease," *Journal of Alzheimer's Disease* 91, no. 1 (2023): 1–23.

17. Lawrence Tabak, "Changes in Human Microbiome Precede Alzheimer's Cognitive Declines," July 26, 2023, https://www.nia.nih .gov/news/changes-human-microbiome-precede-alzheimers-cognitive -declines#:~:text=Earlier%20studies%20showed%20that%20the,before %20any%20obvious%20symptoms%20appear.

18. Z. Li et al., "APOE2: Protective Mechanism and Therapeutic Implications for Alzheimer's Disease," *Molecular Neurodegeneration* 15, no. 63 (2020), https://doi.org/10.1186/s13024-020-00413-4.

19. Berlau et al., "APOE Epsilon2," 2009.

20. Sholpan Askarova et al., "The Links between the Gut Microbiome, Aging, Modern Lifestyle and Alzheimer's Disease," *Frontiers in Cellular and Infection Microbiology* 10 (2020): 104.

21. T. T. T. Tran et al., "*APOE* Genotype Influences the Gut Microbiome Structure and Function in Humans and Mice: Relevance for

Alzheimer's Disease Pathophysiology," *FASEB Journal* 33, no. 7 (2019): 8221–8231, doi: 10.1096/fj.201900071R.

22. "Study Reveals How APOE4 Gene May Increase Risk for Dementia," National Institute on Aging, March 16, 2021, https://www.nia.nih .gov/news/study-reveals-how-apoe4-gene-may-increase-risk -dementia#.

23. Liliana C. Baptista et al., "Crosstalk between the Gut Microbiome and Bioactive Lipids: Therapeutic Targets in Cognitive Frailty," *Frontiers in Nutrition* 7 (2020), https://www.frontiersin.org/articles/10.3389/fnut .2020.00017/full.

24. Payel Kundu et al., "Integrated Analysis of Behavioral, Epigenetic, and Gut Microbiome Analyses in *App*NL-G-F, *App*NL-F, and Wild Type Mice," *Scientific Reports* 11 (2021): 4678, https://www.nature.com /articles/s41598-021-83851-4.

25. Erik Robinson, "Study Finds Changes in Gut Microbiome Connected to Alzheimer's-like Behavior," OHSU News, February 25, 2021, https://news.ohsu.edu/2021/02/25/study-finds-changes-in-gut-micro biome-connected-to-alzheimers-like-behavior#.

26. Ronald D. Hills et al., "Gut Microbiome: Profound Implications for Diet and Disease," *Nutrients* 11, no. 7 (2019): 1613, doi: 10.3390 /nu11071613.

27. Jian Lu, Kun Ling Ma, and Xiong Zhong Ruan, "Dysbiosis of Gut Microbiota Contributes to the Development of Diabetes Mellitus," *Infectious Microbes and Diseases* 1, no. 2 (2019): 43–48, doi: 10.1097 /IM9.0000000000000011.

28. M. Vince, "Meet the Bacteria That Might Help Treat Diabetes," *Medical News Today*, January 7, 2021, https://www.medicalnewstoday .com/articles/meet-the-bacteria-that-might-help-treat-diabetes; R. R. Rodrigues et al., "Transkingdom Interactions between *Lactobacilli* and Hepatic Mitochondria Attenuate Western Diet-Induced Diabetes," *Nature Communications* 12 (2021): 101, https://doi.org/10.1038/s41467 -020-20313-x.

29. Z. Chen et al., "Association of Insulin Resistance and Type 2 Diabetes with Gut Microbial Diversity: A Microbiome-Wide Analysis from Population Studies," *JAMA Network Open* 4, no. 7 (2021): e2118811, doi: 10.1001/jamanetworkopen.2021.18811.

30. "Heart Disease Facts," *CDC*, February 23, 2022, https://www.cdc.gov /heartdisease/facts.htm.

31. G. R. Geovanini and P. Libby, "Atherosclerosis and Inflammation: Overview and Updates," *Clinical Science* 132, no. 12 (2018): 1243–1252, doi: 10.1042/CS20180306.

32. Matej Vicen et al., "Regulation and Role of Endoglin in Cholesterol-Induced Endothelial and Vascular Dysfunction in Vivo and in Vitro," *FASEB Journal* 33, no. 5 (2019): 6099–6114.

CHAPTER 7: CHANGING THE COURSE OF ALZHEIMER'S DISEASE

1. S. Grabrucker et al., "Microbiota from Alzheimer's Patients Induce Deficits in Cognition and Hippocampal Neurogenesis," *Brain* 146, no. 12 (2023): 4916–4934, doi: 10.1093/brain/awad303.

2. Quang Tran, "Gut Health Plays a Role in Alzheimer's Development, New Study Says," Alzheimer's Research UK (March 2, 2022), https://www.alzheimersresearchuk.org/news/gut-health-plays-a-role-in-alzheimers-development-new-study-says/.

3. Aura L. Ferreiro et al., "Gut Microbiome Composition May Be an Indicator of Preclinical Alzheimer's Disease," *Science Translational Medicine* 15, no. 700 (2023): eabo2984, doi: 10.1126/scitranslmed.abo2984.

4. Grabrucker et al., "Microbiota from Alzheimer's Patients," 2023; Quang Tran, "Gut Health Plays a Role in Alzheimer's Development, New Study Says," *Alzheimer's Research UK,* September 28, 2023, https://www.alzheimersresearchuk.org/gut-health-plays-a-role-in-alzheimers-development-new-study-says/.

5. Susan Scott, "New Estimate of Dementia Prevalence Indicates Magnitude of India's Challenge," NIH Fogarty International Center, *Global Health Matters* 22, no. 2 (March/April 2023), https://www.fic.nih.gov/News/GlobalHealthMatters/march-april-2023/Pages/new-estimate-dementia-prevalence-magnitude-india-challenge.aspx.

6. V. Chandra et al., "Prevalence of Alzheimer's Disease and Other Dementias in Rural India: The Indo-US Study," *Neurology* 51, no. 4 (1998): 1000–1008, doi: 10.1212/wnl.51.4.1000.

7. B. Scazzocchio, L. Minghetti, and M. D'Archivio, "Interaction between Gut Microbiota and Curcumin: A New Key of Understanding for the Health Effects of Curcumin," *Nutrients* 12, no. 9 (2020): 2499, doi: 10.3390/nu12092499.

8. Andrea Fairley et al., "Diet Patterns, the Gut Microbiome, and Alzheimer's Disease," *Journal of Alzheimer's Disease* 88, no. 3 (2022): 933–941.

9. Courtney Davis et al., "Definition of the Mediterranean Diet: A Literature Review," *Nutrients* 7, no. 11 (2015): 9139–9153, https://doi.org/10.3390/nu7115459.

10. Chen Wang et al., "Sodium Butyrate Ameliorates the Cognitive Impairment of Alzheimer's Disease by Regulating the Metabolism of Astrocytes." *Psychopharmacology* 239, no. 1 (2022): 1–13.

11. N. Zhu et al., "Claudin-5 Relieves Cognitive Decline in Alzheimer's Disease Mice Through Suppression of Inhibitory GABAergic Neurotransmission," *Aging* 14, no. 8 (2022): 3554–3568, doi: 10.18632/aging.204029.

12. Ioanna Aggeletopoulou et al., "Vitamin D and Microbiome: Molecular Interaction in Inflammatory Bowel Disease Pathogenesis," *American Journal of Pathology* 193, no. 6 (2023): 656–668.

13. Kai Yin and Devendra K. Agrawal, "Vitamin D and Inflammatory Diseases," *Journal of Inflammatory Diseases* 7 (2014): 69–87, doi: 10 .2147/JIR.S63898, https://www.ncbi.nlm.nih.gov/pmc/articles/PMC 4070857/#:~:text=Vitamin%20D%20has%20been%20found,pro inflammatory%20cytokines%20in%20airway%20SMCs.

14. Domenico Plantone et al., "Is There a Role of Vitamin D in Alzheimer's Disease?," *CNS and Neurological Disorders Drug Targets* (epub ahead of print, May 26, 2023), doi: 10.2174/18715273226662305 26164421.

15. Elias Alby, Noushad Padinjakara, and Nicola T. Lautenschlager, "Effects of Intermittent Fasting on Cognitive Health and Alzheimer's Disease," *Nutrition Reviews* 81, no. 9 (2023): 1225–1233, https://doi .org/10.1093/nutrit/nuad021.

16. Alby, Padinjakara, and Lautenschlager, "Effects of Intermittent Fasting," 2023.

17. X. Hu et al., "Intermittent Fasting Modulates the Intestinal Microbiota and Improves Obesity and Host Energy Metabolism," *npj Biofilms and Microbiomes* 9, no. 19 (2023), doi.org/10.1038/s41522 -023-00386-4.

18. Brita Belli, "Yale Researchers Find On-Off Switch for Inflammation Related to Overeating," Yale News, June 29, 2020, https://news.yale .edu/2020/06/29/yale-researchers-find-switch-inflammation-related -overeating.

19. K. Mani, A. Javaheri, and A. Diwan, "Lysosomes Mediate Benefits of Intermittent Fasting in Cardiometabolic Disease: The Janitor Is the Undercover Boss," *Comprehensive Physiology* 8, no. 4 (2018): 1639–1667, doi: 10.1002/cphy.c180005.

20. Mani, Javaheri, and Diwan, "Lysosomes Mediate Benefits," 2018.

21. Mani, Javaheri, and Diwan, "Lysosomes Mediate Benefits," 2018.

22. P. Elwood et al., "Healthy Lifestyles Reduce the Incidence of Chronic Diseases and Dementia: Evidence from the Caerphilly Cohort Study," *PLoS One* 8, no. 12 (2013): e81877, doi: 10.1371/journal.pone.0081877; Nikolaos Scarmeas, Costas A. Anastasiou, and Mary Yannakoulia, "Nutrition and Prevention of Cognitive Impairment," *Lancet Neurology* 17, no. 11 (2018): 1006–1015.

CHAPTER 8: HOW GUT HEALTH CONTRIBUTES TO PARKINSON'S DISEASE

1. A. Planas-Ballve and D. Vilas, "Cognitive Impairment in Genetic Parkinson's Disease," *Parkinson's Disease* 2021 (published online December 30, 2021), doi: 10.1155/2021/8610285. PMID: 35003622;

PMCID: PMC8739522; A. Reeve, E. Simcox, and D. Turnbull, "Ageing and Parkinson's Disease: Why Is Advancing Age the Biggest Risk Factor?," *Ageing Research Reviews* 14, no. 100 (2014): 19–30, doi: 10.1016/j.arr.2014.01.004.

2. Allison W. Williams, "Parkinson Disease in the Elderly Adult," *Missouri Medicine* 110, no. 5 (2013): 406–410, https://www.ncbi.nlm.nih.gov/pmc/articles/PMC6179875/; "What Is Parkinson's?," Parkinson's Europe, February 2018, https://www.parkinsonseurope.org/about-parkinsons/what-is-parkinsons/#:~:text=Parkinson's%20affects%20people%20of%20all,men%20than%20women%20are%20affected.

3. "Understanding Parkinson's," Parkinson's Foundation, accessed December 8, 2023, https://www.parkinson.org/understanding-parkinsons; "Parkinson's Disease: Symptoms and Causes," Mayo Clinic, December 2020, https://www.mayoclinic.org/diseases-conditions/parkinsons-disease/symptoms-causes/syc-20376055.

4. B. A. Killinger and V. Labrie, "Vertebrate Food Products as a Potential Source of Prion-Like α-Synuclein," *NPJ Parkinson's Disease* 3, no. 33 (2017), https://doi.org/10.1038/s41531-017-0035-z.

5. "Lewy Body Dementia (LBD)," Johns Hopkins Medicine, October 29, 2021, https://www.hopkinsmedicine.org/health/conditions-and-diseases/dementia/dementia-with-lewy-bodies.

6. "The Gastrointestinal Tract and Parkinson's," American Parkinson Disease Association, July 17, 2018, https://www.apdaparkinson.org/article/the-gut-and-parkinsons/#:~:text=The%20presence%20of%20Lewy%20bodies,non%2Dmotor%20symptom%20of%20PD.

7. Norihito Uemura et al., "Inoculation of α-Synuclein Preformed Fibrils into the Mouse Gastrointestinal Tract Induces Lewy Body-like Aggregates in the Brainstem via the Vagus Nerve," *Molecular Neurodegeneration* 13, no. 21 (2018), https://molecularneurodegeneration.biomedcentral.com/articles/10.1186/s13024-018-0257-5#:~:text=Braak's%20hypothesis%20based%20on%20autopsy,in%20a%20caudo%2Drostral%20direction.

8. S. K. Dutta et al., "Parkinson's Disease: The Emerging Role of Gut Dysbiosis, Antibiotics, Probiotics, and Fecal Microbiota Transplantation," *Journal of Neurogastroenterology and Motility* 25, no. 3 (2019): 363–376, doi: 10.5056/jnm19044.

9. A. J. Pedrosa Carrasco, L. Timmermann, and D. J. Pedrosa, "Management of Constipation in Patients with Parkinson's Disease," *NPJ Parkinson's Disease* 4, no. 6 (2018), https://doi.org/10.1038/s41531-018-0042-8.

10. A. H. Tan, S. Y. Lim, and A. E. Lang, "The Microbiome-Gut-Brain Axis in Parkinson Disease—From Basic Research to the Clinic," *Nature Reviews Neurology* 18 (2022): 476–495, https://doi.org/10.1038/s41582-022-00681-2.

11. Eamonn M. M. Quigley, "Constipation in Parkinson's Disease," *Seminars in Neurology* 43, no. 4 (2023): 562–571, doi: 10.1055/s-0043 -1771457.

12. Quigley, "Constipation in Parkinson's," 2023; Elizabeth Pennisi, "Meet the Psychobiome," *Science* 368, no. 6491 (2020): 570–573, doi: 10.1126 /science.368.6491.570.

13. Z. S. Agim and J. R. Cannon, "Dietary Factors in the Etiology of Parkinson's Disease," *BioMed Research International* (2015): 672838, doi: 10.1155/2015/672838.

14. M. Alizadeh, S. Kheirouri, and M. Keramati, "What Dietary Vitamins and Minerals Might Be Protective against Parkinson's Disease?," *Brain Sciences* 13, no. 7 (2023): 1119, doi: 10.3390/brainsci13071119.

15. G. Logroscino et al., "Dietary Lipids and Antioxidants in Parkinson's Disease: A Population-Based, Case-Control Study," *Annals of Neurology* 39, no. 1 (1996): 89–94, doi: 10.1002/ana.410390113.

16. Logroscino et al., "Dietary Lipids," 1996.

17. Thomas C. King, *Elsevier's Integrated Pathology* (St. Louis: Mosby, 2007), accessed via https://www.sciencedirect.com/topics/neuroscience /dopaminergic-neuron#:~:text=Parkinson's%20disease%20results%20 from%20loss,14%2D10).

18. M. P. Mattson, "Will Caloric Restriction and Folate Protect Against AD and PD?," *Neurology* 60, no. 4 (2003): 690–695, doi: 10.1212/01 .WNL.0000042785.02850.11.

19. Tan, Lim, and Lang, "The Microbiome-Gut-Brain Axis," 2022.

20. N. Schimelpfening, "Parkinson's Disease May be Caused by Common Dry-Cleaning Chemical," Healthline, March 16, 2023, https://www .healthline.com/health-news/parkinsons-disease-may-be-caused-by -common-dry-cleaning-chemical#:~:text=Scientists%20have%20 proposed%20that%20the,mitochondria%20may%20be%20the%20 cause; Washington State University, "Connection between Household Chemicals and Gut Microbiome," *ScienceDaily,* November 12, 2020, https://www.sciencedaily.com/releases/2020/11/201112080906 .htm.

21. Sarah R. Dash, "The Microbiome and Brain Health: What's the Connection?," Medscape, March 24, 2015, https://www.medscape .com/viewarticle/841748.

CHAPTER 9: CHANGING THE COURSE OF PARKINSON'S DISEASE

1. Kavita R. Gandhi and Abdolreza Saadabadi, "Levodopa (L-Dopa)," StatPearls (Treasure Island, FL, 2024), https://www.ncbi.nlm.nih.gov /books/NBK482140/; Yoshikuni Mizuno, Satoe Shimoda, and Hideki Origasa, "Long-Term Treatment of Parkinson's Disease with Levodopa

and Other Adjunctive Drugs," *Journal of Neurotransmission* 125, no. 1 (January 16, 2018): 35–43, doi: 10.1007/s00702-016-1671-x.

2. X. Sun et al., "Update to the Treatment of Parkinson's Disease Based on the Gut-Brain Axis Mechanism," *Frontiers in Neuroscience* 16 (2022): 878239, doi: 10.3389/fnins.2022.878239.

3. Z. D. Wallen et al., "Metagenomics of Parkinson's Disease Implicates the Gut Microbiome in Multiple Disease Mechanisms," *Nature Communications* 13, no. 6958 (2022), https://doi.org/10.1038/s41467-022-34667-x.

4. Wallen et al., "Metagenomics of Parkinson's," 2022.

5. Wallen et al., "Metagenomics of Parkinson's," 2022.

6. Sarah Vascellari et al., "Clinical Phenotypes of Parkinson's Disease Associate with Distinct Gut Microbiota and Metabolome Enterotypes," *Biomolecules* 11, no. 2 (2021): 144, https://doi.org/10.3390/biom11020144.

7. Z. S. Agim and J. R. Cannon, "Dietary Factors in the Etiology of Parkinson's Disease," *BioMed Research International* (2015): 672838, doi: 10.1155/2015/672838.

8. "Diet & Nutrition," Parkinson's Foundation, accessed March 14, 2024, https://www.parkinson.org/living-with-parkinsons/management/diet-nutrition; Stacy E. Seidl et al., "The Emerging Role of Nutrition in Parkinson's Disease," *Frontiers in Aging Neuroscience* 6 (2014): 36, doi: 10.3389/fnagi.2014.00036.

9. Rosalba Siracusa et al., "Anti-inflammatory and Anti-oxidant Activity of Hidrox in Rotenone-Induced Parkinson's Disease in Mice," *Antioxidants* 9, no. 9 (2020): 824, https://doi.org/10.3390/antiox9090824.

10. Anna Tresserra-Rimbau et al., "Plant-Based Dietary Patterns and Parkinson's Disease: A Prospective Analysis of the UK Biobank," *Movement Disorders* 38, no. 11 (2023): 1994–2004, https://doi.org/10.1002/mds.29580.

11. P. F. Cuevas-González, A. M. Liceaga, and J. E. Aguilar-Toalá, "Postbiotics and Paraprobiotics: From Concepts to Applications," *Food Research International* 136 (2020): 109502, doi: 10.1016/j.foodres.2020.109502; M. Zhu et al., "Gut Microbiota: A Novel Therapeutic Target for Parkinson's Disease," *Frontiers in Immunology* 13 (2022): 937555, doi: 10.3389/fimmu.2022.937555.

12. G. W. Ross et al., "Association of Coffee and Caffeine Intake with the Risk of Parkinson Disease," *Journal of the American Medical Association* 283, no. 20 (2000): 2674-2679, doi: 10.1001/jama.283.20.2674.

13. Brit Mollenhauer and Paul Wilmes, "Dietary Interventions to Slow and Improve Parkinson's Symptoms by Restructuring the Gut Microbiome and Decreasing Inflammation," Michael J. Fox Foundation for

Parkinson's Research, accessed December 17, 2023, https://www
.michaeljfox.org/grant/dietary-interventions-slow-and-improve
-parkinsons-symptoms-restructuring-gut-microbiome-and.

14. Ren Xiangpeng and Jiang-Fen Ren, "Caffeine and Parkinson's Disease: Multiple Benefits and Emerging Mechanisms," *Frontiers in Neuroscience* 14 (2020), doi: 602697. 10.3389/fnins.2020.602697.

15. B. A. Killinger and V. Labrie, "Vertebrate Food Products as a Potential Source of Prion-Like α-Synuclein," *NPJ Parkinson's Disease* 3, no. 33 (2017), https://doi.org/10.1038/s41531-017-0035-z.

16. E. D. Louis et al., "Elevated Blood Harmane (1-methyl-9H-pyrido [3,4-b]indole) Concentrations in Parkinson's Disease," *Neurotoxicology* 40 (2014): 52–56, doi: 10.1016/j.neuro.2013.11.005.

17. C. Anderson et al., "Dietary Factors in Parkinson's Disease: The Role of Food Groups and Specific Foods," *Movement Disorders* 14, no. 1 (1999): 21–27, doi: 10.1002/1531-8257(199901)14:1<21::AID-MDS1006> 3.0.CO;2-Y.

18. H. Chen et al., "Consumption of Dairy Products and Risk of Parkinson's Disease," *American Journal of Epidemiology* 165 (2007): 998–1006, doi: 10.1093/aje/kwk089.

19. O. C. Reddy and Y. D. van der Werf, "The Sleeping Brain: Harnessing the Power of the Glymphatic System through Lifestyle Choices," *Brain Sciences* 10, no. 11 (2020): 868, doi: 10.3390/brainsci 10110868.

20. H. Lee et al., "The Effect of Body Posture on Brain Glymphatic Transport," *Journal of Neuroscience* 35, no. 31 (2015): 11034–11044, https://doi.org/10.1523/jneurosci.1625-15.2015.

21. L. Katz, R. Just, and D. O. Castell, "Body Position Affects Recumbent Postprandial Reflux," *Journal of Clinical Gastroenterology* 18, no. 4 (1994): 280–283, https://doi.org/10.1097/00004836-199406000 -00004.

22. Witoon Mitarnun et al., "Home-Based Walking Meditation Decreases Disease Severity in Parkinson's Disease: A Randomized Controlled Trial," *Journal of Integrative and Complementary Medicine* 28, no. 3 (2022): 227–233.

23. Alice Peck, *Walking with the Seasons: The Wonder of Being in Step with Nature* (London: Ryland Peters & Small, 2024). Adapted with permission of the author.

24. Yanin Machado et al., "Centering Prayer in the Treatment of Parkinson's Disease: Preliminary Quality-of-Life Research," *World Journal of Advanced Research and Reviews* 16, no. 2 (2022): 870–875.

25. Y. Pu et al., "Dietary Intake of Glucoraphanin Prevents the Reduction of Dopamine Transporter in the Mouse Striatum after Repeated Administration of MPTP," *Neuropsychopharmacology Reports* 39, no. 3 (2019): 247–251, doi: 10.1002/npr2.12060.

26. H. L. DuPont et al., "Fecal Microbiota Transplantation in Parkinson's Disease—A Randomized Repeat-Dose, Placebo-Controlled Clinical Pilot Study," *Frontiers in Neurology* 14 (2023): 1104759, doi: 10.3389/fneur.2023.1104759.

27. G. M. Earhart and M. J. Falvo, "Parkinson Disease and Exercise," *Comprehensive Physiology* 3, no. 2 (2013): 833–848, doi: 10.1002/cphy.c100047.

28. Q. Gao et al., "Effects of Tai Chi on Balance and Fall Prevention in Parkinson's Disease: A Randomized Controlled Trial," *Clinical Rehabilitation* 28, no. 8 (2014): 748–753, doi: 10.1177/0269215514521044.

29. Mitarnun et al., "Home-Based Walking Meditation," 2022; Machado et al., "Centering Prayer," 2022.

CHAPTER 10: RECIPES TO HELP CHANGE THE COURSE OF STROKE

1. Fang-yang Huang et al., "Dietary Ginger as a Traditional Therapy for Blood Sugar Control in Patients with Type 2 Diabetes Mellitus," *Medicine (Baltimore)* 98, no. 13 (2019): e15054, doi: 10.1097/MD.0000000000015054.

2. Maki Iizuka et al., "Inhibitory Effects of Balsamic Vinegar on LDL Oxidation and Lipid Accumulation in THP-1 Macrophages," *Journal of Nutritional Science and Vitaminology (Tokyo)* 56, no. 6 (2010): 421–427, doi: 10.3177/jnsv.56.421https://pubmed.ncbi.nlm.nih.gov/21422711/; "Cilantro: 7+ Reasons to Love This Super-Herb for Your Health," Integrative Medicine of New Jersey, accessed March 14, 2024, http://integrativemedicineofnj.com/cilantro-7-reasons-to-love-this-super-herb-for-your-health.

3. H. E. Khoo et al., "Anthocyanidins and Anthocyanins: Colored Pigments as Food, Pharmaceutical Ingredients, and the Potential Health Benefits," *Food and Nutrition Research* 61, no. 1 (2017): 1361779, doi: 10.1080/16546628.2017.1361779.

4. C. Lan et al., "Curcumin Prevents Strokes in Stroke-Prone Spontaneously Hypertensive Rats by Improving Vascular Endothelial Function," *BMC Cardiovascular Disorders* 18, no. 43 (2018), https://doi.org/10.1186/s12872-018-0768-6.

5. Laura Diaz-Marugan et al., "Microbiota, Diet, and the Gut-Brain Axis in Multiple Sclerosis and Stroke," *European Journal of Immunology* 53, no. 11 (2023): 2250229.

6. Kumar Ganesan and Baojun Xu, "Polyphenol-Rich Lentils and Their Health Promoting Effects," *International Journal of Molecular Sciences* 18, no. 11 (2017): 2390, doi: 10.3390/ijms18112390.

7. Aedín Cassidy et al., "Dietary Flavonoids and Risk of Stroke in Women," *Stroke* 43, no. 4 (2012): 946–951.

CHAPTER 11: RECIPES TO HELP CHANGE THE COURSE OF ALZHEIMER'S DISEASE

1. "MIND and Mediterranean Diets Linked to Fewer Signs of Alzheimer's Brain Pathology," *NIH: National Institute on Aging*, May 4, 2023, https://www.nia.nih.gov/news/mind-and-mediterranean-diets-linked-fewer-signs-alzheimers-brain-pathology.

2. José Enrique de la Rubia Ortí et al., "Improvement of Main Cognitive Functions in Patients with Alzheimer's Disease after Treatment with Coconut Oil Enriched Mediterranean Diet: A Pilot Study," *Journal of Alzheimer's Disease* 65, no. 2 (2018): 577–587, doi: 10.3233/JAD-180184.

3. Puja Agarwal et al., "Pelargonidin and Berry Intake Association with Alzheimer's Disease Neuropathology: A Community-Based Study," *Journal of Alzheimer's Disease* 88, no. 2 (2022): 653-661, doi: 10.3233/JAD-215600.

4. University of South Florida, "Natural Compound in Basil May Protect against Alzheimer's Disease Pathology," *Science Daily*, October 5, 2021, www.sciencedaily.com/releases/2021/10/211005101827.htm.

CHAPTER 12: RECIPES TO HELP CHANGE THE COURSE OF PARKINSON'S DISEASE

1. Y. Pu et al., "Dietary Intake of Glucoraphanin Prevents the Reduction of Dopamine Transporter in the Mouse Striatum After Repeated Administration of MPTP," *Neuropsychopharmacology Reports* 39, no. 3 (2019): 247–251, doi: 10.1002/npr2.12060.

2. Anna Tresserra-Rimbau et al., "Plant-Based Dietary Patterns and Parkinson's Disease: A Prospective Analysis of the UK Biobank," *Movement Disorders* 38, no. 11 (2023): 1994–2004, https://doi.org/10.1002/mds.29580.

3. "The Link Between Inflammation & Early Parkinson's," Parkinson's Foundation, August 2, 2023, https://www.parkinson.org/blog/science-news/inflammation#:~:text=New%20research%20suggests%20that%20inflammation,when%20it%20comes%20to%20Parkinson's.

4. Elizabeth Sharpe, "Do Peppers Reduce Risk of Parkinson's?," *UW News*, May 8, 2013, https://www.washington.edu/news/2013/05/08/do-peppers-reduce-risk-of-parkinsons.

5. Rosalba Siracusa et al., "Anti-inflammatory and Anti-oxidant Activity of Hidrox in Rotenone-Induced Parkinson's Disease in Mice," *Antioxidants* 9, no. 9 (2020): 824, https://doi.org/10.3390/antiox9090824.

6. M. Rijntjes, "Knowing Your Beans in Parkinson's Disease: A Critical Assessment of Current Knowledge about Different Beans and Their

Compounds in the Treatment of Parkinson's Disease and in Animal Models," *Parkinson's Disease* (2019): 1349509, doi: 10.1155/2019/134 9509.

GLOSSARY

1. "The Brain-Gut Connection," *John Hopkin's Medicine,* accessed March 14, 2024, https://www.hopkinsmedicine.org/health/wellness-and -prevention/the-brain-gut-connection#:~:text=Scientists%20call%20 this%20little%20brain,tract%20from%20esophagus%20to%20rectum.

INDEX

ABOUT THE AUTHOR

Partha Nandi, MD, FACP, is a gastroenterologist, clinical associate professor of Medicine at Michigan State University, and the chief medical officer and president of Pinnacle GI Partners. He is an international health advocate, keynote speaker, and media expert, whose no-nonsense approach to health and wellness combines Eastern and Western techniques and philosophies. He is also the host of the syndicated television show *The Dr. Nandi Show* with millions of viewers worldwide, the chief health editor at WXYZ ABC Detroit, and the author of the best-selling *Ask Dr. Nandi*. A fellow of the American College of Physicians, he is also an active member of the American Medical Association, the American College of Gastroenterology, the American Gastroenterological Association, and the American Society of Gastrointestinal Endoscopy. Dr. Nandi practices medicine full time in Michigan, where he lives with his wife and children.